A PRACTICAL GUIDE TO **PTSD TREATMENT**

A PRACTICAL GUIDE TO
PTSD TREATMENT

PHARMACOLOGICAL AND PSYCHOTHERAPEUTIC APPROACHES

Edited by Nancy C. Bernardy
and Matthew J. Friedman

American Psychological Association • Washington, DC

Copyright © 2015 by the American Psychological Association. All rights reserved. Except as permitted under the United States Copyright Act of 1976, no part of this publication may be reproduced or distributed in any form or by any means, including, but not limited to, the process of scanning and digitization, or stored in a database or retrieval system, without the prior written permission of the publisher.

Chapters 2, 3, 9, 10, and 11 were coauthored by employees of the United States government as part of official duty and are considered to be in the public domain.

Published by
American Psychological Association
750 First Street, NE
Washington, DC 20002
www.apa.org

To order
APA Order Department
P.O. Box 92984
Washington, DC 20090-2984
Tel: (800) 374-2721; Direct: (202) 336-5510
Fax: (202) 336-5502; TDD/TTY: (202) 336-6123
Online: www.apa.org/pubs/books
E-mail: order@apa.org

In the U.K., Europe, Africa, and the Middle East, copies may be ordered from
American Psychological Association
3 Henrietta Street
Covent Garden, London
WC2E 8LU England

Typeset in Minion by Circle Graphics, Inc., Columbia, MD

Printer: Maple Press, York, PA
Cover Designer: Mercury Publishing Services, Inc., Rockville, MD

The opinions and statements published are the responsibility of the authors, and such opinions and statements do not necessarily represent the policies of the American Psychological Association. Any views expressed in chapters 2, 3, 9, 10, and 11 do not necessarily represent the views of the United States government, and the authors' participation in the work is not meant to serve as an official endorsement.

Library of Congress Cataloging-in-Publication Data

A practical guide to PTSD treatment : pharmacological and psychotherapeutic approaches / [edited by] Nancy C. Bernardy and Matthew J. Friedman. — First edition.
    p. ; cm.
  Includes bibliographical references and index.
  ISBN-13: 978-1-4338-1832-5
  ISBN-10: 1-4338-1832-9
  I. Bernardy, Nancy C., editor. II. Friedman, Matthew J., editor. III. American Psychological Association, issuing body.
  [DNLM: 1. Stress Disorders, Post-Traumatic—drug therapy. 2. Combined Modality Therapy. 3. Psychotherapy—methods. 4. Stress Disorders, Post-Traumatic—therapy. WM 172.5]
  RC552.T7
  616.85′21061—dc23
                                                                2014016420

British Library Cataloguing-in-Publication Data
A CIP record is available from the British Library.

Printed in the United States of America
First Edition

http://dx.doi.org/10.1037/14522-000

Contents

Contributors		vii
Introduction *Nancy C. Bernardy and Matthew J. Friedman*		3
I. Scientific Background and Assessment		**7**
1.	The Human Stress Response *Matthew J. Friedman*	9
2.	The Emerging Scientific and Clinical Literature on Resilience and Psychological First Aid *Steven Southwick and Patricia Watson*	21
3.	Posttraumatic Stress Disorder: Patient Interview, Clinical Assessment, and Diagnosis *Brian P. Marx and Cassidy A. Gutner*	35
II. Pharmacological and Psychotherapeutic Approaches		**53**
4.	Antidepressant Strategies in the Management of PTSD *Nancy C. Bernardy and Matthew J. Friedman*	55
5.	The Use of Anxiolytics in the Management of PTSD *Nancy C. Bernardy, Tasha Souter, and Matthew J. Friedman*	71

CONTENTS

6.	Atypical Antipsychotics and Anticonvulsants in the Treatment of PTSD: Treatment Options That Include Cognitive Behavioral Therapies *Matthew D. Jeffreys*	89
7.	Cognitive Behavioral Therapies for PTSD *Tara E. Galovski and Chelsea Gloth*	101

III. Comorbid Disorders and Unique Presentations — 117

8.	PTSD and Insomnia *Jason C. DeViva and Bruce Capehart*	119
9.	Co-Occurring Substance Use Disorders and PTSD *Andrew J. Saxon and Tracy L. Simpson*	135
10.	Treating PTSD in Older Adults *Joan M. Cook, Ahsan Naseem, and Steven R. Thorp*	151
11.	Challenging Presentations in PTSD *Tonya Masino and Sonya Norman*	163

Index	179
About the Editors	193

Contributors

Nancy C. Bernardy, PhD, National Center for PTSD, VA Medical Center, White River Junction, VT, and The Geisel School of Medicine at Dartmouth, Hanover, NH

Bruce Capehart, MD, OEF/OIF Program, Durham VA Medical Center, and Department of Psychiatry, Duke University, Durham, NC

Joan M. Cook, PhD, Department of Psychiatry, Yale School of Medicine and National Center for PTSD, West Haven, CT

Jason C. DeViva, PhD, Veterans Affairs Connecticut Health Care System, West Haven, and Yale School of Medicine, New Haven, CT

Matthew J. Friedman, MD, PhD, National Center for PTSD, VA Medical Center, White River Junction, VT, and The Geisel School of Medicine at Dartmouth, Hanover, NH

Tara E. Galovski, PhD, Center for Trauma Recovery, Department of Psychology, University of Missouri—St. Louis

Chelsea Gloth, MA, Center for Trauma Recovery, Department of Psychology, University of Missouri—St. Louis

Cassidy A. Gutner, PhD, National Center for PTSD at VA Boston Healthcare System and Department of Psychiatry, Boston University School of Medicine, Boston, MA

Matthew D. Jeffreys, MD, Department of Psychiatry, School of Medicine, The University of Texas Health Science Center at San Antonio

CONTRIBUTORS

Brian P. Marx, PhD, National Center for PTSD at VA Boston Healthcare System and Department of Psychiatry, Boston University School of Medicine, Boston, MA

Tonya Masino, MD, VA San Diego Healthcare System, San Diego, CA

Ahsan Naseem, MD, U.S. Department of Veterans Affairs Nebraska—Western Iowa Health Care System, Omaha

Sonya Norman, PhD, National Center for PTSD and Department of Psychiatry, University of San Diego—California

Andrew J. Saxon, MD, Center of Excellence in Substance Abuse Treatment and Education, VA Puget Sound Health Care System, Seattle, WA

Tracy L. Simpson, PhD, Center of Excellence in Substance Abuse Treatment and Education, VA Puget Sound Health Care System, Seattle, WA

Tasha Souter, MD, VA Palo Alto Health Care System, Palo Alto, and Stanford University School of Medicine, Stanford, CA

Steven Southwick, MD, National Center for PTSD and VA Connecticut Healthcare System, West Haven, and Yale University School of Medicine, New Haven, CT

Steven R. Thorp, PhD, Department of Psychiatry, University of California, San Diego, and VA San Diego Health Care System, San Diego

Patricia Watson, PhD, National Center for PTSD and VA Medical and Regional Office Center, White River Junction, VT

A PRACTICAL GUIDE TO
PTSD TREATMENT

Introduction

Nancy C. Bernardy and Matthew J. Friedman

The validity and clinical utility of the posttraumatic stress disorder (PTSD) diagnosis are now well established after 33 years of scientific testing and clinical use. The PTSD concept reflects an inability to cope with overwhelming stress that is followed by a distinctive pattern of symptoms. It may be most accurate to think of PTSD as a disorder of reactivity in which alterations are best revealed by responses to psychological or pharmacological probes. The PTSD hypothesis has made it possible to develop unique therapeutic approaches, including medications and psychotherapies, that could not have been envisioned without the PTSD model.

The purpose of this book is to translate scientific research on PTSD into testable clinical approaches. By synthesizing the clinical implications of scientific research on PTSD, we hope to provide the rationale for practical clinical strategies that are evidence based. The book is intended to serve as a resource for a broad range of mental health professionals who treat

---

http://dx.doi.org/10.1037/14522-001
A Practical Guide to PTSD Treatment: Pharmacological and Psychotherapeutic Approaches,
N. C. Bernardy and M. J. Friedman (Editors)
Copyright © 2015 by the American Psychological Association. All rights reserved.

patients with PTSD, including primary care providers, psychiatrists, psychologists, social workers, and other clinicians. It is our expectation that the information in this volume will assist clinicians in developing evidence-based and comprehensive treatment plans for their patients with PTSD.

The book covers the existing literature on conventional and novel combination strategies for PTSD treatment. Although our major focus is on pharmacotherapy, we also provide information on the latest research findings on effective psychotherapy approaches. In addition to focusing on treatment of PTSD, we also include information on evidence-based approaches when PTSD is associated with a comorbid disorder (e.g., depression) or significant co-occurring symptoms (e.g., insomnia). Because we designed this book to present evidence from the existing literature on conventional and novel combination therapies for PTSD, we invited leading investigators in the field to present the latest evidence in their respective areas of expertise and to provide a road map for future research.

Part I provides the scientific background for the specific chapters on pharmacotherapy that appear in Part II. It starts with a review of the human stress response in order to provide the psychobiological context in which to understand pharmacological interventions. The next chapter addresses the complex topic of resilience, which includes important genetic and biological components that may stimulate the future development of pharmacological agents. Chapter 3 discusses diagnostic assessment, with specific reference to the diagnostic criteria for PTSD in the new fifth edition of the *Diagnostic and Statistical Manual of Mental Disorders*.

Part II provides an overview of pharmacological and other treatments for PTSD. It includes separate chapters on antidepressants, anxiolytics, and antipsychotics. Chapter 4 provides an overview of antidepressants, which currently constitute first-line recommended evidence-based pharmacological treatments for PTSD. Chapter 5 follows with a review of medications that decrease anxiety, one of the major symptoms of PTSD, with a primary focus on benzodiazepines and why their use should be minimized. Chapter 6 then focuses on less commonly used medications—antipsychotics and anticonvulsants—with a review of the mixed evidence regarding their efficacy and information regarding side effects. These pharmacological chapters are followed in Chapter 7 by an overview of the latest information on cognitive–behavioral psychotherapies for PTSD that includes information about what is known about the combination of pharmacotherapy and psychotherapy.

Part III provides information on co-occurring conditions with PTSD. This section includes chapters that address treatment of specific symptoms that require clinical attention, such as insomnia (Chapter 8) and substance use (Chapter 9), as well as treatment of older adults (Chapter 10) and those with complicated clinical presentations (Chapter 11).

We have tried to be as rigorous and comprehensive as possible while recognizing that the answers to many important questions regarding the best choice of treatment require additional research. In addition to clinical trials to determine the efficacy of different treatments, we need more research to help us understand both the pathophysiology of PTSD and the mechanisms of action of effective therapeutic approaches. For example, on the basis of research on depression (Forgeard et al., 2011), it seems likely that cognitive–behavioral therapy for PTSD is mediated by top-down, neocortical mechanisms through which the prefrontal cortex exerts restraint on the amygdala. Similarly, it seems likely that medications have a bottom-up, subcortical action by directly targeting the amygdala, hippocampus, locus coeruleus, raphe nuclei, and other key areas of the brain. However, the truth is that more research is needed before we can make such statements conclusively. We also need to know where and how different medications exert their beneficial effects and whether different psychotherapeutic approaches work in different ways. Trials that compare the recommended cognitive–behavioral therapy approaches such as prolonged exposure or cognitive processing therapy need to be compared with eye movement desensitization or present-centered therapy to determine not only relative efficacy but also how these different psychotherapies ameliorate PTSD. Information is also needed on predictors of treatment outcome. Some patients may be better candidates for psychotherapy, whereas others may be better candidates for medication.

New directions in the field for pharmacotherapy are also needed. The current medications in use were all initially designed to treat other disorders (e.g., antidepressants, antihypertensives, anticonvulsants, antipsychotics). There is a clear need for medications that preferentially target the abnormal psychobiological mechanisms associated with PTSD. There is also a great need for research on augmentation strategies for partial responders to evidence-based pharmacotherapy as well as on treatments for PTSD and co-occurring conditions. Furthermore, there is a serious shortage of randomized clinical trials of safe, effective medications for children. Finally, there is always the question about the generalizability of results from published clinical trials to cohorts that may not have been well represented in such trials; for example, questions remain about the applicability of the current evidence base to children, older individuals, and people from different ethnocultural settings.

The good news is that more effective treatment options are now available for our patients than ever before. Despite this, we still need much more research to address important questions for which solid evidence is lacking. As we move to a shared decision-making model in which patients participate in discussions with providers about different treatment options, clinicians need not only to be well informed about recommended evidence-based treatments but also to recognize what isn't known, at present, because the current research is inconclusive.

We hope that you find this book useful and that it provides helpful guidance as you confront the challenges of treating individuals with PTSD.

REFERENCE

Forgeard, M. J. C., Haigh, E. A. P., Beck, A. T., Davidson, R. J., Henn, F. A., Maier, S. F., . . . Seligman, M. E. P. (2011). Beyond depression: Towards a process-based approach to research, diagnosis and treatment. *Clinical Psychology: Science and Practice, 18*, 275–299. doi:10.1111/j.1468-2850.2011.01259.x

ONE

SCIENTIFIC BACKGROUND AND ASSESSMENT

1

The Human Stress Response
Matthew J. Friedman

The human stress response is an elegant and complex psychobiological system of reactions that has evolved for coping, adaptation, and survival of the species. At its core, it is built around the capacity for rapid recognition of potentially harmful stimuli to mobilize the species-specific defense response (SSDR; see Figure 1.1; Shalev, Gilboa, & Rasmusson, 2011). The basolateral nucleus of the amygdala (BLA) processes afferent sensory and visceral information regarding threatening stimuli. Once activated, basolateral neurons project to the central nucleus of the amygdala, which instigates and coordinates the key components of the SSDR. These include autonomic (e.g., cardiovascular, respiratory), neuroendocrine (e.g., hypothalamic–pituitary–adrenocortical [HPA] axis), skeletal muscle (e.g., fight, flight, or freeze behaviors), and changes in information processing (e.g., overgeneralization of threat) behaviors. The central nucleus of the amygdala projects directly to brainstem monoaminergic nuclei such

http://dx.doi.org/10.1037/14522-002
A Practical Guide to PTSD Treatment: Pharmacological and Psychotherapeutic Approaches,
N. C. Bernardy and M. J. Friedman (Editors)
Copyright © 2015 by the American Psychological Association. All rights reserved.

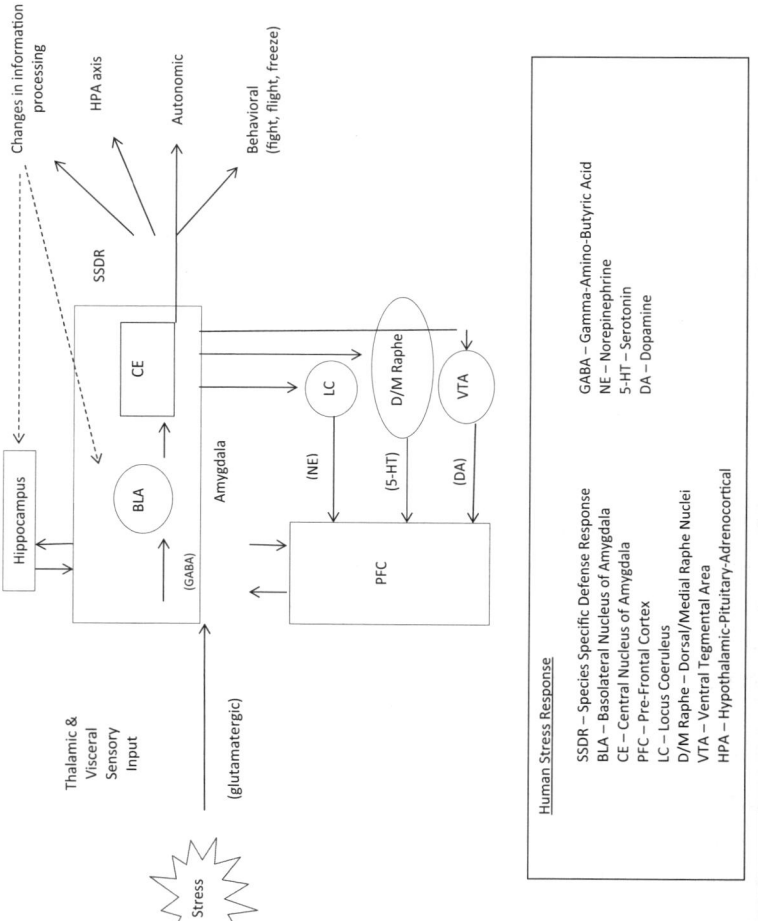

Figure 1.1.

The species-specific defense response showing key brain structures and neurotransmitters that mediate the SSDR. From "Biological Studies of Post-Traumatic Stress Disorder," by R. K. Pitman, A. M. Rasmusson, K. C. Koenen, L. M. Shin, S. P. Orr, M. W. Gilbertson, M. R. Milad, and I. Liberzon, 2012, *Nature Reviews Neuroscience, 13*, p. 778. Copyright 2012 by Nature Publishing Group. Adapted with permission.

as the ventral tegmental area, locus coeruleus, and medial and dorsal raphe nuclei that activate dopamine (DA), norepinephrine (NE), and serotonin (5-HT), respectively. As a result, these monoamines play an important role in modulating the SSDR (Pitman et al., 2012).

The prefrontal cortex (PFC) is the key component of the SSDR that provides top-down control of emotional responses and amygdalar restraint. The PFC has multiple regions (including dorsolateral PFC, medial PFC, orbitofrontal cortex, and anterior cingulate). It also regulates the nucleus accumbens, which is a key reward region of the brain (Feder, Nestler, & Charney, 2009; Nash, Galatzer-Levy, Krystal, Duman, & Neumeister, 2014). At moderate or manageable stress levels, glutamatergic pyramidal output neurons from the PFC tonically activate inhibitory (gamma-aminobutyric acid [GABA]-ergic) neurons within the BLA, which in turn suppress central nucleus activation of the SSDR. During intense stress, however, excessive NE output suppresses PFC restraint on the amygdala, thereby igniting unrestrained amygdala activation of the SSDR (Pitman et al., 2012; Shalev et al., 2011). DA and 5-HT, acting at DA and 5-HT$_{24}$ receptors, contribute to this amygdala storm by suppressing glutamatergic stimulation of inhibitory GABA-ergic neurons within the BLA. Because the BLA is more primitive (e.g., paleocortex), its processing power is limited and less nuanced than other brain structures involved in the SSDR. As a result, it tends to respond to extreme stress with "precipitous and 'all-or-none' qualities of defensive reactions experienced during traumatic stress and in PTSD [posttraumatic stress disorder]" (Shalev et al., 2011, p. 96). Indeed, the BLA's threat-appraisal bias is toward false positives because a false negative threat can harm or kill an individual.

The hippocampus is the third major brain structure to consider with respect to the SSDR. It provides contextual information about the circumstances under which the SSDR has been activated in the past, thereby contributing to threat appraisal by the BLA. In concert with the PFC, the hippocampus calibrates and modulates amygdalar response to incoming sensory information (Nash et al., 2014; Pitman et al., 2012).

Exposure to threatening situations activates fear conditioning. The excessive outpouring of NE during the SSDR facilitates the encoding of fearful memories associated with the traumatic event (Pitman et al., 2012;

Rasmusson & Shalev, 2014; Shalev et al., 2011). Such heightened information processing leads to fear conditioning in which threat cues (e.g., unconditioned stimuli) become consolidated within amygdala circuits, and associated cues also become consolidated (as conditioned stimuli) within a classic Pavlovian paradigm. This is clearly adaptive because survival may depend on the capacity to remember dangerous experiences in order to avoid or prepare for them in the future. It is not adaptive, however, to activate the SSDR when there is no danger or the danger has passed, as is the case with specific phobias, PTSD, or anxiety disorders. This is the rationale for adaptation of laboratory fear extinction paradigms for clinical use, as with prolonged exposure therapy for PTSD. Another treatment, cognitive processing therapy, has been shown (with functional magnetic resonance imaging) to decrease amygdalar activation and to increase PFC activation; indeed, lateral PFC activation is associated with reappraisal success (Goldin et al., 2008).

There are individual differences regarding threat appraisal and subsequent mobilization of the SSDR. Research on resilience indicates that many factors contribute to such differences, including genetic, experiential, psychosocial, and characterological factors; coping capacity; social competence; and the perception of life as meaningful (Feder et al., 2009; Southwick, Litz, Charney, & Friedman, 2011; see also Chapter 2, this volume). Among these, research on candidate genes related to PTSD is especially exciting. More than 20 candidate genes have been identified. As might be expected, they moderate a number of key systems involved in the SSDR, such as adrenergic, dopaminergic, serotonergic, HPA, GABAergic, and other mechanisms (see Koenen et al., 2014; Pitman et al., 2012).

NEUROTRANSMITTERS, NEUROPEPTIDES, AND NEUROHORMONES

To consider potential pharmacological interventions, it is necessary to know how various neurotransmitters, neuropeptides, and neurohormones mediate and moderate the SSDR. In the following sections, we review such mechanisms.

Norepinephrine

NE has been identified as a key neurotransmitter mediating the SSDR since the classic work of Walter Cannon (1932), who recognized that the sympathetic nervous system and adrenal gland were involved in the fight-or-flight response to threat. Eighty years later, we understand that key brain adrenergic mechanisms mediate the SSDR. Mild and manageable stress increases adrenergic input to high-affinity alpha-2 receptors in the PFC. This facilitates fine discrimination of environmental sensory input in conjunction with experiential memories stored in the hippocampus and with PFC working memory. The convergence of all this relevant information permits "executive decision making and guidance of behavior" at a time that amygdala activity is tonically inhibited by the PFC through glutamatergic inputs that activate inhibitory intra-amygdala GABA-ergic interneurons (Rasmusson & Shalev, 2014; Shalev et al., 2011).

At higher stress levels, increased adrenergic input activates low-affinity alpha-1 receptors. (DA and $5HT-2_A$ receptors are also synergistically activated at the same time.) The result is that PFC function is greatly impaired, especially with respect to working memory and amygdalar restraint (Arnsten, 2009). Under such conditions, BLA function reverts to a more primitive, less informed, and less nuanced status so that the amygdala's central nucleus activation is more likely to be triggered by conditioned stimuli (e.g., neutral cues associated with unconditional threat cues) and the BLA response is more likely to be a primitive precipitous, "all-or-none" reaction, as noted previously. Concurrently, amygdala GABA-ergic and other inhibitory activity is diminished in conjunction with a major reduction in PFC restraint. It is a "perfect storm" with excessive amygdala activity unleashed from PFC and GABA-ergic control.

Dopamine

DA contributes to activation of the SSDR through two actions in the BLA. DA (D_1) receptors reduce PFC-induced glutamatergic inhibition of BLA activity. In addition, DA (D_2) receptors promote increased BLA responsivity to sensory inputs. Taken together, these mechanisms promote conditioned fear responding, contribute to stress generalization, and enhance behaviors such as hypervigilance and sensitivity to environmental cues (Rasmusson & Shalev, 2014).

Serotonin

There are many 5-HT receptors that have different actions. For example, activation of 5-HT_{1A} receptors is anxiolytic, whereas 5-HT_{2A} receptors are anxiogenic and potentiate the SSDR during extreme stress (along with NE and DA). Furthermore, meta-chlorophenylpiperazine, which acts at many 5-HT receptors but especially at the 5-HT_{2B} and 5-HT_{2C} receptors, precipitates panic attacks and PTSD flashbacks among veterans with PTSD (Rasmusson & Shalev, 2014). Finally, 5-HT_{2C} receptors are involved in fear-related freezing behavior (Kennett et al., 1994). Thus, the 5-HT_2 receptor class appears to promote the SSDR and fear response (Charney, 2004; Rasmusson & Shalev, 2014). The conflicting actions of 5-HT_2 and 5-HT_{1A} receptors may, at least partially, account for the limited efficacy of selective serotonin reuptake inhibitors in PTSD (Friedman, 2013).

Corticotropin-Releasing Hormone

Corticotropin-releasing hormone (CRH) is one of the most important components of the SSDR. It activates arousal and fear behaviors as well as locus coeruleus–based adrenergic input. Activation of CRH in response to stress initiates the HPA component of the SSDR. As a hypothalamic hormone, CRH promotes secretion of adrenocorticotropin from the pituitary, which promotes release of glucocorticoids, such as cortisol and dehydroepiandrosterone, from the adrenal cortex. In addition to these neuroendocrine effects, CRH-containing neurons are located in a number of key nuclei involved in the SSDR, such as the PFC (including the cingulate cortex), central nucleus of the amygdala, locus coeruleus, and raphe nuclei. Mobilization of amygdalar CRH neurons activates fear-related behaviors. CRH-1 and CRH-2 receptors have opposite actions; CRH-1 receptors promote anxiety and stress intolerance, whereas CRH-2 receptors are anxiolytic (Charney, 2004).

Cortisol and Dehydroepiandrosterone

Cortisol and dehydroepiandrosterone (DHEA) are secreted synchronously as a major component of the HPA response. Cortisol acts synergistically with NE to mobilize energy, increase arousal, focus attention, and potentiate memory formation and fear learning (Charney, 2004). Whereas acute cortisol release is an important component of the SSDR, chronic cortisol dysregulation, as seen in chronic stress or PTSD, can have serious medical and psychiatric effects (Friedman & McEwen, 2004). DHEA and its sulfated derivative DHEAS oppose many actions of cortisol, including protection against cortisol-mediated neurotoxicity, regulation of apoptosis (e.g., programmed cell death), and promotion of neurogenesis in the hippocampus (Charney, 2004; Rasmusson & Shalev, 2014). DHEA also antagonizes GABA receptors, thereby facilitating fear conditioning and fear extinction through *N*-methyl-D-aspartate mediated activity. Research with U.S. special forces personnel exposed to extreme stress indicates that DHEA is associated with improved performance and resilience (Morgan, Rasmusson, Pietrzak, Coric, & Southwick, 2009).

Neuropeptide Y

Neuropeptide Y (NPY) is colocated with adrenergic neurons distributed throughout the brain, sympathetic nervous system, and adrenal medulla. Presynaptic NPY-Y2 autoreceptors restrain neuronal excitation, whereas postsynaptic NPY-Y1 receptors potentiate NE activity. In the amygdala, NPY-Y1 receptors have an anxiolytic activity that opposes CRH-induced anxiogenesis. In the hippocampus, NPY-Y1 receptors promote neurogenesis that protects against cortisol-induced neurotoxicity (Charney, 2004; Rasmusson & Shalev, 2014). As with DHEA, NPY is positively associated with resilience, improved performance, and enhanced PFC function among U.S. special forces exposed to extreme stress (Morgan et al., 2002). NPY also promotes recovery from stress-induced energy depletion (Rasmusson & Shalev, 2014).

Allopregnanolone and Pregnanolone

Allopregnanolone and its equipotent enantiomer pregnanolone are neuroactive steroids known collectively as ALLO. ALLO is a powerful and selective modulator of GABA action at $GABA_A$ receptors. Acute stress increases ALLO levels, which exert a tonic inhibitory influence on stress-related excitation. It is noteworthy that ALLO produces such inhibition at benzodiazepine-resistant $GABA_A$ receptors. With regard to the SSDR, ALLO provides negative feedback on HPA activity. Behaviorally, it exerts anxiolytic, sedative, neuroprotective, and regenerative effects. Finally, there is evidence that selective serotonin reuptake inhibitors' antidepressant therapeutic effects are mediated through ALLO activation (Pinna, Costa, & Guidotti, 2009; Rasmusson & Shalev, 2014).

Immune Factors

There are strong functional relationships between the immune system and other components of the SSDR (Baker, Nievergelt, & O'Connor, 2012; Najjar, Pearlman, Alper, Najjar, & Devinsky, 2013). Glucocorticoids and catecholamines inhibit the production of proinflammatory cytokines such as interleukin (IL)-1 beta, IL-6, and IL-12, tumor necrosis factor-alpha, and interferon-gamma. They also stimulate production of anti-inflammatory cytokines such as IL-10, IL-4, and transforming growth factor-beta (Elenkov & Chrousos, 2002). There is some suggestion that such acute immunological reactions are associated with negative mood states. This area of research is only beginning to receive the attention it deserves.

RELEVANCE TO PTSD

The psychobiology of the SSDR provides the necessary context for understanding PTSD and psychobiological resilience. Mobilization of the SSDR is adaptive and resilient when the response is sufficient to cope with the present threat but is terminated as soon as the danger has passed. In PTSD, however, it appears that many components of the SSDR have been sustained and remain in effect. Such a chronic prolongation of these mechanisms has deleterious long-range effects. For example, the neurocircuitry of PTSD is characterized by excessive amygdala activation and reduced PFC and hippocampal activity, as in the SSDR. There is excessive NE, reduced NPY, and adrenergic dysregulation in PTSD. HPA dysregulation is also evident with elevated CRH and glucocorticoid upregulation. With regard to serotonin, $5\text{-}HT_2$ receptor expression appears to be increased at the expense of $5\text{-}HT_{1A}$ receptor function. ALLO and DHEA/DHEAS expression appears to be diminished. Finally, elevations in proinflammatory cytokines and chemokines have been detected (Charney, 2004; Feder et al., 2009; Friedman & McEwen, 2004; Hoge et al., 2009; Nash et al., 2014; Pitman et al., 2012; Rasmusson & Shalev, 2014).

IMPLICATIONS FOR INTERVENTION AND TREATMENT

The best way to prevent most cases of PTSD is to eliminate manmade traumas such as war, rape, genocide, and abusive violence. Because that does not appear to be likely in the foreseeable future, enhancing resilience and implementing widespread public mental health preventive measures is the next-best option. With regard to helping individuals who have been exposed to a traumatic event, interventions must be calibrated to optimize the SSDR by preventing excessive and maladaptive expression of the human stress response; such interventions must also terminate the response when it is no longer effective and adaptive (e.g., a "morning after pill"; M. J. Friedman, 2002). Finally, we can expect that the most effective treatments for PTSD will reduce the allostatic load produced by the maladaptive chronic perpetuation of the human stress response.

REFERENCES

Arnsten, A. F. (2009). Stress signalling pathways that impair prefrontal cortex structure and function. *Nature Reviews Neuroscience, 10*, 410–422. doi:10.1038/nrn2648

Baker, D. G., Nievergelt, C. M., & O'Connor, D. T. (2012). Biomarkers of PTSD: Neuropeptides and immune signaling. *Neuropharmacology, 62*, 663–673. doi:10.1016/j.neuropharm.2011.02.027

Cannon, W. B. (1932). *The wisdom of the body*. New York, NY: Norton.

Charney, D. S. (2004). Psychobiological mechanisms of resilience and vulnerability: Implications for successful adaptation to extreme stress. *The American Journal of Psychiatry, 161*, 195–216. doi:10.1176/appi.ajp.161.2.195

Elenkov, I. J., & Chrousos, G. P. (2002). Stress hormones, proinflammatory and antiinflammatory cytokines, and autoimmunity. *Annals of the New York Academy of Sciences, 966*, 290–303. doi:10.1111/j.1749-6632.2002.tb04229.x

Feder, A., Nestler, E. J., & Charney, D. S. (2009). Psychobiology and molecular genetics of resilience. *Nature Reviews Neuroscience, 10*, 446–457. doi:10.1038/nrn2649

Friedman, M. J. (2002). Future pharmacotherapy for post-traumatic stress disorder: Prevention and treatment. *Psychiatric Clinics of North America, 25*, 427–441. doi:10.1016/S0193-953X(02)00010-2

Friedman, M. J. (2013). PTSD: Pharmacotherapeutic approaches. *Focus, 11*, 315–320.

Friedman, M. J., & McEwen, B. S. (2004). Posttraumatic stress disorder, allostatic load, and medical illness. In P. P. Schnurr & B. L. Green (Eds.), *Trauma and health: Physical health consequences of exposure to extreme stress* (pp. 157–188). Washington, DC: American Psychological Association. doi:10.1037/10723-007

Goldin, P. R., McRae, K., Ramel, W., & Gross, J. J. (2008). The neural bases of emotion regulation: Reappraisal and suppression of negative emotion. *Biological Psychiatry, 63*, 577–586. doi:10.1016/j.biopsych.2007.05.031

Hoge, E. A., Brandstetter, K. A., Moshier, S., Pollack, M. H., Wong, K.-K., & Simon, N. M. (2009). Broad spectrum of cytokine abnormalities in panic disorder and posttraumatic stress disorder. *Depression and Anxiety, 26*, 447–455. doi:10.1002/da.20564

Kennett, G. A., Lightowler, S., De Biasi, V., Stevens, N. C., Wood, M. D., Tulloch, I. F., & Blackburn, T. P. (1994). Effect of chronic administration of selective 5-hydroxytryptamine and noradrenaline uptake inhibitors on a putative index of 5-HT2C2B receptor function. *Neuropharmacology, 33*, 1581–1588. doi:10.1016/0028-3908(94)90133-3

Koenen, K. C., Guffanti, G., Yan, L., Haloossim, M., Uddin, M., Nugent, N., & Amstadter, A. (2014). The genetics of posttraumatic stress disorder. In M. J. Friedman, T. M. Keane, & P. A. Resick (Eds.), *Handbook of PTSD: Science and practice* (2nd ed., pp. 300–312). New York, NY: Guilford Press.

Morgan, C. A., III, Rasmusson, A., Pietrzak, R. H., Coric, V., & Southwick, S. M. (2009). Relationships among plasma dehydroepiandrosterone and dehydroepiandrosterone sulfate, cortisol, symptoms of dissociation, and objective performance in humans exposed to underwater navigation stress. *Biological Psychiatry, 66,* 334–340. doi:10.1016/j.biopsych.2009.04.004

Morgan, C. A., III, Rasmusson, A. M., Wang, S., Hoyt, G., Hauger, R. L., & Hazlett, G. (2002). Neuropeptide-Y, cortisol, and subjective distress in humans exposed to acute stress: replication and extension of previous report. *Biological Psychiatry, 52,* 136–142. doi:10.1016/S0006-3223(02)01319-7

Najjar, S., Pearlman, D. M., Alper, K., Najjar, A., & Devinsky, O. (2013). Neuroinflammation and psychiatric illness. *Journal of Neuroinflammation, 10,* 43. doi:10.1186/1742-2094-10-43

Nash, M., Galatzer-Levy, T., Krystal, J. H., Duman, R., & Neumeister, A. (2014). Neurocircuitry and neuroplasticity in PTSD. In M. J. Friedman, T. M. Keane, & P. A. Resick (Eds.), *Handbook of PTSD: Science and practice* (2nd ed., pp. 251–274). New York, NY: Guilford Press.

Ochsner, K. N., Ray, R. D., Cooper, J. C., Robertson, E. R., Chopra, S., Gabrieli, J. D., & Gross, J. J. (2004). For better or for worse: Neural systems supporting the cognitive down- and up-regulation of negative emotion. *NeuroImage, 23,* 483–499. doi:10.1016/j.neuroimage.2004.06.030

Pinna, G., Costa, E., & Guidotti, A. (2009). SSRIs act as selective brain steroidogenic stimulants (SBSSs) at low doses that are inactive on 5-HT reuptake. *Current Opinion in Pharmacology, 9,* 24–30. doi:10.1016/j.coph.2008.12.006

Pitman, R. K., Rasmusson, A. M., Koenen, K. C., Shin, L. M., Orr, S. P., Gilbertson, M. W., . . . Liberzon, I. (2012). Biological studies of post-traumatic stress disorder. *Nature Reviews Neuroscience, 13,* 769–787. doi:10.1038/nrn3339

Rasmusson, A. M., & Shalev, A. (2014). Integrating the neuroendocrinology, neurochemistry and neuroimmunology of PTSD to date and the challenges ahead. In M. J. Friedman, T. M. Keane, & P. A. Resick (Eds.), *Handbook of PTSD: Science and practice* (2nd ed., pp. 275–299). New York, NY: Guilford Press.

Shalev, A., Gilboa, A., & Rasmusson, A. M. (2011). Neurobiology of stress, trauma, and PTSD. In D. J. Stein, M. J. Friedman, & C. Blanco (Eds.), *Trauma and mental health: Resilience and posttraumatic stress disorders* (pp. 89–138). West Sussex, England: Wiley.

Southwick, S. M., Litz, B. T., Charney, D., & Friedman, M. J. (Eds.). (2011). *Resilience and mental health: Challenges across the lifespan.* Cambridge, England: Cambridge University Press. doi:10.1017/CBO9780511994791

2

The Emerging Scientific and Clinical Literature on Resilience and Psychological First Aid

Steven Southwick and Patricia Watson

This chapter begins by defining *resilience* and then describes the neurobiological and psychosocial factors that are associated with it. This is followed by a discussion of possible strategies to enhance resilience. The chapter ends with comments on potential ways to reduce the probability of developing trauma-related psychopathology.

Resilience is generally understood as the ability to bend but not break and to bounce back from adversity. An individual's ability to manage and flourish under high levels of stress has far-reaching implications for physical and mental health. Chronic stress that is poorly managed can contribute to a host of illnesses, such as heart disease, diabetes, gastric ulcers, and depression. On the other hand, the ability to modulate the stress response and

---

This chapter was coauthored by employees of the United States government as part of official duty and is considered to be in the public domain. Any views expressed herein do not necessarily represent the views of the United States government, and the authors' participation in the work is not meant to serve as an official endorsement.

http://dx.doi.org/10.1037/14522-003
A Practical Guide to PTSD Treatment: Pharmacological and Psychotherapeutic Approaches,
N. C. Bernardy and M. J. Friedman (Editors)
Copyright © 2015 by the American Psychological Association. All rights reserved.

bounce back from traumas and setbacks can be protective and even growth promoting. The American Psychological Association (2010) defined *resilience* as "the process of adapting well in the face of adversity, trauma, tragedy, threats or even significant sources of threat."

In recent years, researchers have attempted to understand and define resilience more systematically. This has been challenging because resilience is a complex construct with individuals typically handling stress more effectively in some domains of their life (e.g., work) compared with other domains (e.g., interpersonal relationships). In addition, individuals may be more resilient during some phases of their life (e.g., middle age) than during other phases (e.g., adolescence; Southwick, Litz, Charney, & Friedman, 2011). Currently, a number of assessment instruments are used to measure resilience, including the Connor Davidson Scale (Connor & Davidson, 2003), the Response to Stressful Experiences (Johnson et al., 2011), and the Dispositional Resilience Scales (Bartone, 2007).

FACTORS THAT INFLUENCE RESILIENCE

Understanding resilience is also complex because the manner in which someone handles stress and trauma is influenced by many factors, including genetic, neurobiological, developmental, psychological, and social factors.

Genetic Factors

Genetic factors clearly play an important role in behavior and in responses to stress. For example, it has been estimated that overall heritability of posttraumatic stress disorder (PTSD) ranges from 32% to 38% (True et al., 1993). Studies examining how variations in specific genes affect the stress response and resilience are of great interest but thus far have led to few replicable findings. Stress researchers have been particularly interested in gene variants that affect the noradrenergic, dopamine, serotonin, and hypothalamic–pituitary–adrenocortical (HPA) axis systems (DiGangi, Guffanti, McLaughlin, & Koenen, 2013). For example, most, but not all, genetic studies of the serotonin system have found that individuals who inherit a high expression variant of the serotonin transporter gene exhibit less activation of the amygdala when viewing aversive or fearful stimuli and are less likely to develop depression after a major life stress compared with individuals who inherit a low expression variant (Caspi, Hariri, Holmes, Uher, & Moffitt, 2010). In recent years it has become increasingly clear that environmental stimuli, both internal (e.g., stress, fear) and external (e.g., social support, drug use), can trigger biochemical reactions that either activate or silence genes (Toyokawa, Uddin, Koenen, & Galea, 2012).

Developmental Factors

The manner in which one is raised has an important impact on later ability to manage stress. Repetitive exposure to overwhelming and uncontrollable stress and trauma, such as child abuse, has been linked with exaggerated sympathetic nervous system, HPA axis, and behavioral responses to future stresses in adolescence and adulthood. In contrast, repetitive childhood exposure to mild to moderate stress that the child can handle and master may have a stress inoculating or "steeling" affect, meaning that future neurobiological and behavioral responses to stress are less robust and better modulated than normal (Lyons, Parker, & Schatzberg, 2010; Southwick et al., 2011).

Neurobiological Factors

Chronic failure to effectively modulate the stress response can impair the immune system, damage neurons in the hippocampus and prefrontal cortex, and contribute to a host of psychological and medical conditions, including depression, anxiety, asthma, and heart disease.

The biology of resilience likely involves a complex network of brain circuits associated with emotion regulation, response to fear, social behavior, learning, memory, extinction, and reward. On the basis of a large body of animal research and emerging research in humans, it has been suggested that resilience may be related to (a) well-modulated sympathetic nervous system and HPA axis responses to stress that are characterized by rapid activation and rapid return to baseline once the stress has subsided; (b) functional hippocampi that provide sufficient inhibition to the HPA axis and that can adequately differentiate safe from dangerous environments; (c) robust prefrontal cortical function and inhibition of limbic, behavioral, and emotional responses to stress and fear; (d) amygdala activity that is well regulated and that does not overrespond to stress and fear; and (e) a dopamine-mediated reward system that is durable, remains functional, and fosters positive emotions even under situations of chronic stress (Feder, Haglund, Wu, Southwick, & Charney, 2013).

Psychosocial Factors

Numerous psychosocial factors have been associated with resilience. In most cases, it is not fully known whether and to what degree these factors are simply associated with resilience or actually promote it. Commonly cited resilience-related psychosocial factors include positive emotions and realistic optimism; the ability to regulate emotions; active as opposed to passive coping style; disciplined focus on skill development; an attitude in which stress is viewed as a potential opportunity for growth, and challenges are typically met head-on and overcome whenever possible; regular exercise and good physical fitness; a strong social support network; cognitive flexibility with the tendency to accept that which cannot be changed and the ability to reframe adversity in a more positive light; adherence to a set of valued moral and ethical principles; altruism; an active spiritual-religious practice; high coping self-efficacy; and commitment to a valued and meaningful mission, cause, or purpose (Bonanno, Westphal, & Mancini, 2011; Hobfoll, 2001; Southwick, Vythilingam, & Charney, 2005).

Community Factors

Some communities are more resilient to a variety of stressors than others. Norris and colleagues have developed a model of community resilience that includes four primary sources of strength: economic development, social capital, information and communication, and community competence

(Norris, Stevens, Pfefferbaum, Wyche, & Pfefferbaum, 2008). In this model, community resilience is fostered when citizens actively participate in community affairs, are emotionally connected to common concerns and values of the community, work together to solve problems with creativity and flexibility, effectively communicate with one another, invest in a broad range of resources, and share their resources.

NEUROBIOLOGICAL AND PHARMACOLOGICAL STRATEGIES TO ENHANCE RESILIENCE

To date, little is known about the neurobiology of resilience. To develop pharmacological interventions to enhance resilience and reduce the likelihood of developing trauma-related psychopathology, researchers must continue to conduct both animal and human investigations into mechanisms involved in activation and modulation of the stress response. On the basis of what is currently known, a number of potential neurobiologically based resilience-enhancing interventions have been proposed. For example, animal and human studies suggest that excessive and prolonged arousal after exposure to a traumatic event may damage the body and brain and increase the likelihood of developing trauma-related psychopathology (Dohrenwend & Dohrenwend, 1974; Kendler, Karkowski, & Prescott, 1999; Monat, Lazarus, & Reevy, 2007). It has been hypothesized that administering agents that modulate arousal by regulating the sympathetic nervous system and the HPA axis within an optimal level and duration of activation would serve a protective role. Potential candidates include neuropeptide Y, corticotropin-releasing hormone antagonists, dehydroepiandrosterone, and other agents that help to balance excitatory and inhibitory brain processes (Morgan, Krystal, & Southwick, 2003). Antidepressants have also been suggested because they are known to stimulate regrowth of hippocampal neurons (Duman & Monteggia, 2006) that have been damaged by stress and because they have been shown to protect against learned helplessness in animals. To help reduce the overconsolidation of traumatic memories and possible reexperiencing symptoms of PTSD, a number of agents have been proposed, including beta-blockers and morphine (Pitman et al., 2002). Pharmacologic agents might also be used to help modulate neural pathways that are involved in regulating emotional responses to stress and fear, facilitating extinction of traumatic memories, increasing and sustaining positive emotions, enhancing adaptive social behaviors, and promoting recovery from stress.

PSYCHOSOCIAL TRAINING TO ENHANCE RESILIENCE

There are a growing number of programs and strategies for high-risk populations that aim to promote overall wellness and psychological health, as well as prevent PTSD, most notably in the military sector. An example of one such program is Comprehensive Soldier and Family Fitness (CSF), an initiative that seeks to assess and train soldiers and families to achieve more "psychological strength" to thrive and to meet a wide range of operational demands. It does so by focusing on strengthening physical resilience (through exercise, nutrition, and training), emotional resilience (by promoting self-control, stamina, and a responsible and optimistic approach to life challenges), social resilience (through the development and maintenance of trusted, valued relationships and friendships), spiritual resilience (through the development of purpose, core values, beliefs, identity, and life vision), and family resilience (by fostering safe, supportive, and loving family relations). However, Steenkamp, Nash, and Litz (2013) pointed out that more research is needed on resilience-building programs like CSF because the CSF program evaluation findings show small differences between CSF and control conditions. These authors argued that good leadership, morale, cohesion, and training have consistently been associated with lower PTSD scores and represent potentially important avenues to wellness promotion and disorder prevention, as the Navy and Marine Corps Combat and Operational Stress First Aid model hopes to achieve (Nash & Watson, 2012).

Two additional well-known resilience training programs are Hardiness Training and Stress Inoculation Training (SIT). Hardiness Training, which has demonstrated efficacy in dealing with a variety of difficult situations among adults and college students, was designed to foster attitudes of control (i.e., the belief that the trainee can influence events in life), commitment (i.e., feeling deeply involved in the self and one's existence, activities, and relationships), and challenge (i.e., viewing adverse events as challenges; Khoshaba & Maddi, 2001). SIT, which has demonstrated efficacy in lowering state-anger levels in female assault victims, was developed to foster attitudes that are associated with resilience. As part of the training, a variety of coping skills are taught, including relaxation training, guided self-dialogue, thought stopping, problem solving, identification and replacement of maladaptive and irrational thinking, and imaging and behavioral rehearsal (Cahill, Rauch, Hembree, & Foa, 2003; Meichenbaum & Deffenbacher, 1988). Military and first responder trainings that are patterned on stress inoculation principles typically include scenario-based exercises that gradually expose the trainee to a wide range of progressively more challenging cognitive, physical, and emotional skills associated with resilience.

In addition to more comprehensive training programs such as CSF, Hardiness Training, and SIT, there are a host of training programs or interventions that are designed to enhance specific factors associated with resilience. Examples include the following: Learned Optimism, a cognitive behavioral approach to fostering positive emotions (Seligman, 1991), has been shown to reduce symptoms of anxiety and depression in those who completed a training workshop compared with participants in a control group (Seligman, Schulman, DeRubeis, & Hollon, 1999). Network Support Therapy, designed to improve the extent and quality of one's social network (Litt, Kadden, Kabela-Cormier, & Petry, 2007), has been shown to foster self-efficacy and coping in changing drinking behaviors (Litt, Kadden, Kabela-Cormier, & Petry, 2009). Mindfulness meditation training has been associated with improved ability to focus attention, greater flexibility of thinking, increased capacity to cope with anxiety and depression, enhanced psychological well-being, and increased activation of the left prefrontal cortex, which is associated with an increase in positive emotions and more rapid recovery from feelings of anger and fear (Davidson & McEwen, 2012; Kabat-Zinn, 1990).

EARLY INTERVENTION

Although first responders and military service members typically receive some sort of training to foster resilience, they often do not seek formal support in the early aftermath of potentially traumatic stress, and civilians with high exposure to trauma and loss in disasters are often neither trained ahead of time nor do they seek formal mental health intervention. Thus, after a traumatic event, Stress First Aid and Psychological First Aid models have been developed for first responder and civilian populations to provide assistance in obtaining practical and social resources, as well as support to maintain or reestablish the ability to respond flexibly to the demands of the situation. These models, although not yet empirically supported, aim to promote recovery from adversity and stress by instilling hope and promoting a sense of safety, calm, connectedness, and self- and community efficacy, the five essential elements that are consistently related to recovery after adversity and traumatic stress (Hobfoll et al., 2007; Shultz & Forbes, 2013).

Highly affected individuals may require more potent cognitive behavioral interventions that target risk and vulnerability factors and reinforce naturally occurring protective factors in a number of ways, such as assistance in problem solving and acquiring practical resources, setting achievable goals, managing stress reactions, mastering fear around trauma-related situations and activities, and engaging in cognitive reappraisal and restructuring that help redefine appraisals and beliefs in more adaptive ways (Bryant, Moulds, & Nixon, 2003; Nash & Watson, 2012; Rothbaum et al., 2012). Even in situations of ongoing threat, it has been shown that individuals can learn to recognize the benefits of accepting a certain level of risk to permit optimal functioning (Bryant et al., 2011). In this way, cognitive behavioral techniques appear to enhance resilience and help to prevent subsequent psychopathology when delivered in the early phase following a traumatic stressor (Bisson & Cohen, 2006; Roberts, Kitchiner, Kenardy, & Bisson, 2009).

Cognitive behavioral interventions may be effective for a number of reasons related to resilience. For instance, although their primary purpose is to directly address cognitive and behavioral risk factors, which gives the client a sense of choice and control, such interventions also create a structure that decreases the clients' sense of being overwhelmed, help them focus on what they can do in the present moment, and give them a positive sense of self-efficacy as they learn to cope with the aftermath of adversity and traumatic stress. Finally, the provider and client create a partnership or collaboration that makes the client feel supported. Cognitive behavioral techniques are also focused on building skills that give people a sense of having the resources to address the difficulties they may encounter.

There is still a great need for research that will evaluate the effectiveness of early intervention strategies in a number of contexts and eventually evaluate the effectiveness of each separate component, especially with respect to the optimal timing of such interventions. Programs will also need to find more effective ways to increase the acceptability and likelihood that individuals who are highly affected by trauma will engage in more formal treatment in early phases after traumatic stress and adversity (Brewin et al., 2010; Shalev et al., 2012).

CONCLUSION

Resilience is a complex construct that is influenced by a host of genetic, developmental, neurobiological, and psychological factors, as well as by one's relationships, community, available resources, culture, and religious and spiritual life. Progress has been made in both targeting resilience factors and in promoting resilience and recovery in high-risk populations, but research is still needed to determine the most effective, efficient, and acceptable programs for fostering resilience in a broad array of populations and contexts, as well as the optimal time frames for implementing resilience-enhancing interventions.

REFERENCES

American Psychological Association. (2010). *The road to resilience*. Retrieved from http://www.apa.org/helpcenter/road-resilience.aspx

Bartone, P. T. (2007). Test–retest reliability of the Dispositional Resilience Scale—15, a brief hardiness scale. *Psychological Reports, 101*, 943–944. doi:10.2466/pr0.101.3.943-944

Bisson, J. I., & Cohen, J. A. (2006). Disseminating early interventions following trauma. *Journal of Traumatic Stress, 19,* 583–595. doi:10.1002/jts.20175

Bonanno, G. A., Westphal, M., & Mancini, A. D. (2011). Resilience to loss and potential trauma. *Annual Review of Clinical Psychology, 7,* 511–535. doi:10.1146/annurev-clinpsy-032210-104526

Brewin, C. R., Fuchkan, N., Huntley, Z., Robertson, M., Thompson, M., Scragg, P., ... Ehlers, A. (2010). Outreach and screening following the 2005 London bombings: Usage and outcomes. *Psychological Medicine, 40,* 2049–2057.

Bryant, R. A., Ekassawin, S., Chakkraband, M. L. S., Suwanmitri, S., Duangchun, O., & Chantaluckwong, T. (2011). A randomized controlled effectiveness trial of cognitive behavior therapy for post-traumatic stress disorder in terrorist-affected people in Thailand. *World Psychiatry; Official Journal of the World Psychiatric Association, 10,* 205–209.

Bryant, R. A., Moulds, M. L., & Nixon, R. V. D. (2003). Cognitive behaviour therapy of acute stress disorder: A four-year follow-up. *Behaviour Research and Therapy, 41,* 489–494. doi:10.1016/S0005-7967(02)00179-1

Cahill, S. P., Rauch, S. A. M., Hembree, E. A., & Foa, E. B. (2003). Effect of cognitive-behavioral treatments for PTSD on anger. *Journal of Cognitive Psychotherapy, 17,* 113–131. doi:10.1891/jcop.17.2.113.57434

Caspi, A., Hariri, A. R., Holmes, A., Uher, R., & Moffitt, T. E. (2010). Genetic sensitivity to the environment: The case of the serotonin transporter gene and its implications for studying complex diseases and traits. *The American Journal of Psychiatry, 167,* 509–527. doi:10.1176/appi.ajp.2010.09101452

Connor, K. M., & Davidson, J. R. (2003). Development of a new resilience scale: The Connor-Davidson Resilience Scale (CD-RISC). *Depression and Anxiety, 18,* 76–82. doi:10.1002/da.10113

Davidson, R. J., & McEwen, B. S. (2012). Social influences on neuroplasticity: Stress and interventions to promote well-being. *Nature Neuroscience, 15,* 689–695. doi:10.1038/nn.3093

DiGangi, J., Guffanti, G., McLaughlin, K. A., & Koenen, K. C. (2013). Considering trauma exposure in the context of genetics studies of posttraumatic stress disorder: A systematic review. *Biology of Mood & Anxiety Disorders, 3,* 2.

Dohrenwend, B. S., & Dohrenwend, B. P. (Eds.). (1974). *Stressful life events: Their nature and effects.* New York, NY: Wiley.

Duman, R. S., & Monteggia, L. M. (2006). A neurotrophic model for stress-related mood disorders. *Biological Psychiatry, 59,* 1116–1127. doi:10.1016/j.biopsych.2006.02.013

Feder, A., Haglund, M., Wu, G., Southwick, S., & Charney, D. (2013). *The Neurobiology of resilience* (4th ed.). New York, NY: Oxford University Press.

Hobfoll, S. E. (2001). The Influence of Culture, Community, and the Nested-Self in the Stress Process: Advancing Conservation of Resources Theory. *Applied Psychology: An International Review, 50,* 337–421. doi:10.1111/1464-0597.00062

Hobfoll, S. E., Watson, P. J., Bell, C. C., Bryant, R. A., Brymer, M. J., Friedman, M. J., ... Ursano, R. J. (2007). Five essential elements of immediate and midterm mass trauma intervention: Empirical evidence. *Psychiatry: Interpersonal and Biological Processes, 70,* 283–315.

Johnson, D. C., Polusny, M. A., Erbes, C. R., King, D., King, L., Litz, B. T., ... Southwick, S. M. (2011). Development and initial validation of the Response to Stressful Experiences Scale. *Military Medicine, 176,* 161–169. doi:10.7205/MILMED-D-10-00258

Kabat-Zinn, J. (1990). *Full catastrophe living: Using the wisdom of your body and mind to face stress, pain, and illness.* New York, NY: Delacorte Press.

Kendler, K. S., Karkowski, L. M., & Prescott, C. A. (1999). Causal relationship between stressful life events and the onset of major depression. *The American Journal of Psychiatry, 156,* 837–841.

Khoshaba, D. M., & Maddi, S. R. (2001). *HardiTraining: A comprehensive approach to mastering stressful circumstances* (3rd ed.). Newport Beach, CA: Hardiness Institute.

Litt, M. D., Kadden, R. M., Kabela-Cormier, E., & Petry, N. (2007). Changing network support for drinking: Initial findings from the Network Support Project. *Journal of Consulting and Clinical Psychology, 75,* 542–555. doi:10.1037/0022-006X.75.4.542

Litt, M. D., Kadden, R. M., Kabela-Cormier, E., & Petry, N. (2009). Changing network support for drinking: Network Support Project 2-year follow-up. *Journal of Consulting and Clinical Psychology, 77,* 229–242. doi:10.1037/a0015252

Lyons, D. M., Parker, K. J., & Schatzberg, A. F. (2010). Animal models of early life stress: Implications for understanding resilience. *Developmental Psychobiology, 52,* 616–624. doi:10.1002/dev.20500

Meichenbaum, D. H., & Deffenbacher, J. L. (1988). Stress inoculation training. *The Counseling Psychologist, 16,* 69–90. doi:10.1177/0011000088161005

Monat, A., Lazarus, R. S., & Reevy, G. (Eds.). (2007). *The Praeger handbook on stress and coping* (Vol. 1). Westport, CT: Praeger.

Morgan, C. A., III, Krystal, J. H., & Southwick, S. M. (2003). Toward early pharmacological posttraumatic stress intervention. *Biological Psychiatry, 53,* 834–843. doi:10.1016/S0006-3223(03)00116-1

Nash, W. P., & Wattson, P. J. (2012). Review of VA/DOD Clinical Practice Guideline on management of acute stress and interventions to prevent posttraumatic stress disorder. *Journal of Rehabilitation, Research, and Development, 49*, 637–48.

Norris, F. H., Stevens, S. P., Pfefferbaum, B., Wyche, K. F., & Pfefferbaum, R. L. (2008). Community resilience as a metaphor, theory, set of capacities, and strategy for disaster readiness. *American Journal of Community Psychology, 41*, 127–150. doi:10.1007/s10464-007-9156-6

Pitman, R. K., Sanders, K. M., Zusman, R. M., Healy, A. R., Cheema, F., Lasko, N. B., . . . Orr, S. P. (2002). Pilot study of secondary prevention of posttraumatic stress disorder with propranolol. *Biological Psychiatry, 51*, 189–192. doi:10.1016/S0006-3223(01)01279-3

Roberts, N. P., Kitchiner, N. J., Kenardy, J., & Bisson, J. I. (2009). Systematic review and meta-analysis of multiple-session early interventions following traumatic events. *The American Journal of Psychiatry, 166*, 293–301.

Rothbaum, B. O., Kearns, M. C., Price, M., Malcoun, E., Davis, M., Ressler, K. J., . . . Houry, D. (2012). Early intervention may prevent the development of posttraumatic stress disorder: A randomized pilot civilian study with modified prolonged exposure. *Biological Psychiatry, 72*, 957–963. doi:10.1016/j.biopsych.2012.06.002

Seligman, M. E. P. (1991). *Learned optimism.* New York, NY: Knopf.

Seligman, M. E. P., Schulman, P., DeRubeis, R. J., & Hollon, S. D. (1999). The prevention of depression and resilience to stress: Implications for prevention and treatment. *Annual Review of Clinical Psychology, 1*, 255–291.

Shalev, A. Y., Ankri, Y. L. E., Israeli-Shalev, Y., Peleg, T., Adessky, R. S., & Freedman, S. A. (2012). Prevention of posttraumatic stress disorder by early treatment: Results from the Jerusalem trauma outreach and prevention study. *Archives of General Psychiatry, 69*, 166–176. doi:10.1001/archgenpsychiatry.2011.127

Shultz, J. M., & Forbes, D. (2013). Psychological first aid: Rapid proliferation and the search for evidence. *Disaster Health, 1*, 1–10.

Southwick, S. M., Litz, B. T., Charney, D., & Friedman, M. J. (Eds.). (2011). *Resilience and mental health: Challenges across the lifespan.* Cambridge, England: Cambridge University Press. doi:10.1017/CBO9780511994791

Southwick, S. M., Vythilingam, M., & Charney, D. S. (2005). The psychobiology of depression and resilience to stress: Implications for prevention and treatment. *Annual Review of Clinical Psychology, 1*, 255–291. doi:10.1146/annurev.clinpsy.1.102803.143948

Steenkamp, M. M., Nash, W. P., & Litz, B. T. (2013). Post-traumatic stress disorder: Review of the Comprehensive Soldier Fitness program. *American Journal of Preventive Medicine, 44*, 507–512.

Toyokawa, S., Uddin, M., Koenen, K. C., & Galea, S. (2012). How does the social environment "get into the mind"? Epigenetics at the intersection of social and psychiatric epidemiology. *Social Science & Medicine, 74,* 67–74. doi:10.1016/j.socscimed.2011.09.036

True, W. R., Rice, J., Eisen, S. A., Heath, A. C., Goldberg, J., Lyons, M. J., & Nowak, J. (1993). A twin study of genetic and environmental contributions to liability for posttraumatic stress symptoms. *Archives of General Psychiatry, 50,* 257–264. doi:10.1001/archpsyc.1993.01820160019002

3

Posttraumatic Stress Disorder: Patient Interview, Clinical Assessment, and Diagnosis

Brian P. Marx and Cassidy A. Gutner

Although the vast majority of the population is exposed to traumatic stress at some point in life, only a relatively small percentage of exposed individuals develop posttraumatic stress disorder (PTSD; Ozer, Best, Lipsey, & Weiss, 2003). Research has identified a number of pre-, peri-, and posttraumatic factors that contribute to an individual's failure to recover naturally after a trauma. Pretrauma factors that increase risk for PTSD include female gender; younger age at the time of stressor exposure; racial or ethnic minority status (Brewin, Andrews, & Valentine, 2000; Ozer et al., 2003); previous trauma exposure (Delahanty, Raimonde, Spoonster, & Cullado, 2003; King, King, Foy, & Gudanowski, 1996; Nishith, Mechanic, & Resick, 2000); a family history of psychiatric problems (Breslau, Davis, Andreski, &

This chapter was coauthored by an employee of the United States government as part of official duty and is considered to be in the public domain. Any views expressed herein do not necessarily represent the views of the United States government, and the author's participation in the work is not meant to serve as an official endorsement.

http://dx.doi.org/10.1037/14522-004
A Practical Guide to PTSD Treatment: Pharmacological and Psychotherapeutic Approaches,
N. C. Bernardy and M. J. Friedman (Editors)
Copyright © 2015 by the American Psychological Association. All rights reserved.

Peterson, 1991); psychopathology before trauma (e.g., Blanchard, Hickling, Taylor, & Loos, 1995; Bromet, Sonnega, & Kessler, 1998); dysfunction in the family of origin, such as childhood abuse or family instability (Andrews, Brewin, Rose, & Kirk, 2000; King et al., 1996); and genetic vulnerability (e.g., Cornelis, Nugent, Amstadter, & Koenen, 2010). Peritraumatic risk factors for PTSD include trauma severity, perceived threat of injury or death (e.g., King, King, Gudanowski, & Vreven, 1995; King, King, Salgado, & Shalev, 2003), peritraumatic dissociation (e.g., Ozer et al., 2003), intense emotional responses (e.g., shame, guilt, generalized fear; Ozer et al., 2003), and exposure to grotesque events (e.g., Kessler, Sonnega, Bromet, Hughes, & Nelson, 1995). Finally, research has shown that posttrauma social support, or lack thereof, is associated with PTSD (Ozer et al., 2003).

This chapter describes common risk factors for PTSD and some of the changes to the PTSD diagnostic criteria for the fifth edition of the *Diagnostic and Statistical Manual of Mental Disorders* (*DSM–5;* American Psychiatric Association, 2013). We also review some of the available self-report questionnaires and diagnostic interviews that clinicians can use in a thorough evaluation of stressor exposure, PTSD symptoms, and associated functional impairment. Recommendations are made about when to use each measure, as well as how to interpret responses to inform clinical decisions.

PTSD DIAGNOSTIC CRITERIA

In the fourth edition, text revision, of the *DSM* (*DSM–IV–TR;* American Psychiatric Association, 2000), PTSD was classified as in the Anxiety Disorder category. In the *DSM–IV–TR*, to be diagnosed with PTSD, an individual needed to be exposed to an event that involved either actual or threatened death or serious injury or a threat to the physical integrity of oneself or others and resulted in the individual feeling either intense fear, helplessness, or horror (stressor criterion also known as Criterion A in the *DSM–IV–TR*). In addition, the individual was required to experience at least one reexperiencing symptom (Criterion B; e.g., intrusive thoughts, nightmares), three avoidance and numbing symptoms (Criterion C; e.g., avoidance of thoughts, feeling, places, experience feelings of detachment), and two hyperarousal symptoms (Criterion D; e.g., sleep difficulties, exaggerated startle) for at least 30 days (Criterion E). In addition, these symptoms must result in clinically significant distress or dysfunction (Criterion F).

For the *DSM–5* (American Psychiatric Association, 2013), the PTSD committee revised the PTSD diagnostic criteria in several important ways. Specifically, PTSD has been moved from the Anxiety Disorders into a new category, Trauma and Stressor-Related Disorders. The stressor criterion (Criterion A) now places greater emphasis on the temporal relationship between the event and the other symptoms and reframes *DSM–IV–TR*'s indirect or secondhand exposure (i.e., hearing about a trauma from another source instead of directly experiencing or witnessing it) as traumatic only when the information is about a close relative or friend, when (in the case of a fatality) the death is violent or accidental, or when the exposure did not occur via media (e.g., television), unless it is part of one's job. Because past research has found that PTSD Criterion A2 in *DSM–IV–TR* (i.e., the presence of peritraumatic fear, helplessness, or horror in response to a stressor) was not sufficiently predictive of the development of PTSD (see Bovin & Marx, 2011), the committee removed this criterion from the diagnosis. The PTSD symptom clusters have also been somewhat reorganized. The first symptom cluster (Criterion B) remains largely unchanged in terms of the symptoms included but is now labeled Intrusion Symptoms to highlight the intrusive nature of these symptoms. The second symptom cluster (Criterion C), now labeled Persistent Avoidance of Stimuli Associated With Traumatic Event(s), consists of two effortful avoidance symptoms that were previously included with both avoidance and numbing symptoms in PTSD symptom cluster C of *DSM–IV–TR*. The third symptom cluster (Criterion D) includes symptoms (many of which were cluster C "numbing" symptoms in *DSM–IV–TR*) that are now designated as Negative Alterations in Cognitions and Mood That Are Associated With the Traumatic Event. This new category contains new symptom criteria that reflect persistent negative appraisals and pervasive negative mood and emphasizes specific deficits in the capacity to experience positive emotions. The fourth symptom cluster (previously the D Arousal cluster in *DSM–IV–TR*) has been relabeled Alterations in Arousal and Reactivity That Are Associated With the Traumatic Event. It comprises symptoms related to changes in arousal and reactivity and includes irritable and aggressive behavior as well as a new symptom, reckless or self-destructive behavior.

Initial research suggests that the *DSM–5* revisions to the PTSD diagnostic criteria may not substantially alter the expected prevalence of the disorder. For example, Miller et al. (2013) found that, in a national sample of 2,953 participants who completed an online survey, the presumed prevalence of PTSD using the *DSM–5* criteria was 16.6% for lifetime PTSD and 9.1% for PTSD in the past 12 months, whereas the presumed prevalence of PTSD in this same sample using the *DSM–IV–TR* diagnostic criteria was 16.4% for lifetime PTSD and 9.8% for PTSD in the past 12 months. In a separate sample of 345 veterans who completed the same questionnaires either online or via postal survey, Miller et al. found that the presumed prevalence of PTSD using the *DSM–5* criteria was 75.2% for lifetime PTSD and 38.7% for current PTSD, whereas the presumed prevalence of PTSD in this same sample using the *DSM–IV–TR* diagnostic criteria was 74.0% for lifetime PTSD and 39.9% for current PTSD. Results from this study also confirmed the four-cluster *DSM–5* structure of PTSD. In another study, Calhoun et al. (2012) found that the *DSM–5* PTSD criteria showed good concordance with the *DSM–IV–TR* PTSD criteria in a sample of 185 participants recruited from two medical centers. Of particular note, this study showed that slightly fewer participants met *DSM–5* Criterion A (89%) than *DSM–IV–TR* Criterion A (95%). The authors suggested that this difference may have resulted in a slight decrease in prevalence rates.

The 11th edition of the *International Classification of Diseases* (*ICD-11*) is planned for approval by the World Health Assembly in 2015 (Maercker et al., 2013) and proposes to determine a diagnosis of PTSD through a combination of PTSD symptoms falling under three categories. The diagnosis would require at least one reexperiencing symptom (requiring flashbacks and/or nightmares), one avoidance symptom (avoidance of internal and/or external trauma cues), and one or more symptoms of heightened threat and arousal (hypervigilance and/or exaggerated startle). To meet criteria for PTSD under the *ICD–11*, symptoms would need to be present for several weeks and cause significant functional impairment (Maercker et al., 2013).

EVALUATION OF PTSD SYMPTOMS

A number of psychometrically sound self-report and interview measures have been developed to assess the presence and severity of trauma exposure and the cardinal symptoms of PTSD (for a more comprehensive review, see Bovin & Weathers, 2012). Self-report instruments provide a time-efficient method of assessing current symptoms and can easily be administered more frequently to provide weekly information regarding current functioning. Clinician-administered diagnostic interviews take more time to administer than self-report measures and usually yield better quality data but also typically require training. Notably, both self-report scales and interview-based assessment methods are vulnerable to response biases and memory failures; as a result, reliance on a single instrument may lead to an inaccurate diagnosis. To avoid this, we recommend that clinicians use multiple methods and measures to better inform diagnostic decisions (Weathers, Keane, & Foa, 2009). An assessment approach that includes self-report questionnaires, clinician-administered diagnostic interviews, and behavioral observations takes advantage of each method's relative strengths, overcoming the psychometric limitations of any single instrument and maximizing correct diagnostic decisions. However, because individual patient's needs are different and determine the evaluation procedures to be used accordingly, each of these components may not always be used in every assessment case.

Trauma Exposure Measures

Several reliable and valid trauma exposure measures have been created to assess a range of traumatic events. The Life Events Checklist (LEC; Blake et al., 1995) is a commonly used instrument to screen for trauma exposure that can be used in conjunction with diagnostic interviews such as the Clinician Administered PTSD Scale (CAPS; Weathers et al., 2012) or as a standalone instrument. The LEC asks respondents whether they ever experienced, witnessed, or learned about 16 potential events (e.g., natural disasters, sexual assault, combat exposure). The Traumatic Life Events Questionnaire (Kubany et al., 2000) is another well-known self-report trauma exposure measure that assesses a wide range of events. Respondents are asked to indicate how many times they experienced each type of event, from *never* to *more than 5 times* and whether fear, helplessness, or horror was present. The final question of the measure has the patient identify the event endorsed that results in the most distress, the age at which it first occurred and last occurred, and the amount of distress (*no distress* to *extreme distress*) that resulted from the event. Other commonly used self-report measures of trauma exposure include the Trauma History Questionnaire (Green, 1996) and the Traumatic Events Questionnaire (Vrana & Lauterbach, 1994).

The Deployment Risk and Resilience Inventory—2 (DRRI–2; Vogt, Smith, King, & King, 2012) is a measure comprising 17 individual scales that assess risk and resilience factors related to predeployment (e.g., childhood stress), deployment (e.g., combat experiences, perceived threat, harassment), and postdeployment (e.g., social support, family functioning) for active duty military personnel and veterans. Although the DRRI–2 was developed for research, in a clinical setting, its scales can be used to foster a discussion between the patient and therapist about traumatic experiences and the impact they have had as a means to better understand the effects of their experience on both mental and physical health.

For a comprehensive and detailed assessment of lifetime trauma exposure, clinicians can use the Evaluation of Lifetime Stressors (ELS; Krinsley, Gallagher, Weathers, Kaloupek, & Vielhauer, 1997). The ELS is an assessment protocol for adolescents or adults comprising a 56-item self-report questionnaire and 56-item semistructured interview. The questionnaire assesses exposure to traumatic experiences using four response options ("Yes, I can remember this"; "I'm not sure if this happened"; "No, but this happened to someone else in my family"; and "No, this did not happen"). The 56-item interview is organized into nine modules (some optional) that examine questionnaire responses using specific probe questions. The interview explores various dimensions of each trauma (e.g., trauma type, duration, frequency, perceptions of threats, emotional response). Finally, using in-depth querying interview, clinicians can assess the worst two or three events in terms of other dimensions such as dissociation, disclosure, and treatment.

Self-Report PTSD Symptom Measures

Mental health professionals can use self-report measures of PTSD to screen for the disorder. Screening in primary care and other settings offers an opportunity to identify trauma-exposed individuals with undiagnosed or subsyndromal PTSD and intervene as soon as possible. Some of the most widely used screening instruments include the Primary Care Posttraumatic Stress Disorder screen (versions reflecting *DSM–IV–TR* and *DSM–5* interpretations of the disorder are available [Prins et al., 2004]; a version reflecting *DSM–5* diagnostic criteria is currently in development), the Startle Physiological Arousal, Anger and Numbness Scale (Meltzer-Brody, Churchill, & Davidson, 1999), the Short Screening Scale for PTSD (Breslau, Peterson, Kessler, & Schultz, 1999), and the Short Posttraumatic Stress Disorder Rating Interview (Connor & Davidson, 2001). These scales are all relatively brief (between four and 10 items) and have good psychometric properties.

In some cases, it might be beneficial to use a self-report measure that covers all of the symptoms of PTSD because that might provide a better sense of whether an individual actually meets diagnostic criteria for the disorder. Some examples of these measures are the PTSD Checklist, or PCL, for *DSM–IV–TR* and *DSM–5*, the Posttraumatic Stress Diagnostic Scale (PDS), and the Davidson Trauma Scale (Davidson et al., 1997). The PCL (Weathers, Litz, Herman, Huska, & Keane, 1993) has been used extensively with military, civilian, and veteran samples and demonstrates excellent reliability and validity (e.g., McDonald & Calhoun, 2010; Wilkins, Lang, & Norman, 2011). The PCL has been updated to reflect the changes to the diagnostic criteria in *DSM–5* (PCL–5; Weathers et al., 2010). The psychometrics of the PCL–5 are currently being evaluated. The PCL and PCL–5 can be administered relatively quickly, providing clinicians an ideal tool to provide additional information during assessment and then weekly during the course of treatment. Each of the items on the PCL and PCL–5 corresponds directly to the *DSM–IV–TR* and *DSM–5* PTSD diagnostic criteria, respectively, and can be anchored to a specific traumatic event. Respondents rate the extent to which each symptom bothers them on a 5-point scale (1 = *not at all*, 5 = *extremely*). For both the PCL and PCL–5, item scores are summed to create an overall PTSD symptom severity score. Likewise, for both new and old versions, a presumptive PTSD diagnosis can be rendered using several approaches: (a) determining whether an individual meets *DSM* symptom criteria for the various items (i.e., symptoms rated as *moderately* or above are counted as present), (b) determining whether the total severity score exceeds a given cutpoint, or (c) combining methods (a) and (b) to ensure that an individual has sufficient severity as well as the necessary pattern of symptoms required by the *DSM* (e.g., Hoge et al., 2004). Preliminary data suggest that a score of 38 may be used as a cutoff for presumptive PTSD on the PCL–5.

The PCL for *DSM–IV–TR* has also been used to assess symptom severity at weekly and monthly intervals in the clinical setting to monitor symptom change over the course of treatment. In this context, a 5- to 10-point change on the PCL represents reliable change, and a 10-point drop indicates a clinically significant change (Monson et al., 2008). If a clinician does not begin to see a change in the PCL during treatment, it can provide additional information about what the patient might be struggling with (e.g., avoidance of situations, avoidance of trauma triggers) that might be less obvious than something like not completing homework assignments.

In addition to the PCL and PCL–5, there are other well-validated measures of PTSD symptoms from which to choose, including the Posttraumatic Dialogistic Scale (Foa, Cashman, Jaycox, & Perry, 1997). Like the PCL, the PDS is a *DSM*-correspondent measure with four sections: (a) a trauma checklist, (b) a space to provide a written description of the traumatic event, (c) items that correspond to all PTSD symptomatology, and (d) degree of symptom interference. Other well-known validated self-report measures of

PTSD symptoms include the Mississippi Scale for Combat-Related PTSD (Keane, Caddell, & Taylor, 1988), the Impact of Events Scale—Revised (Weiss & Marmar, 1996), the Symptom Checklist 90—Revised (Derogatis, 1994), and the PK Scale of the Minnesota Multiphasic Personality Inventory—2 (Keane, Malloy, & Fairbanks, 1984).

PTSD Diagnostic Interview Measures

Like the PCL, the CAPS (Weathers, Keane, & Davidson, 2001) has been used extensively with various trauma-exposed samples, can be used to assess both current and lifetime PTSD, and demonstrates excellent reliability and validity (e.g., Weathers et al., 2001). Recently, the CAPS was updated to reflect the changes to the PTSD diagnostic criteria in *DSM–5* (CAPS–5; Weathers et al., 2012). Psychometrics of the CAPS–5 are currently undergoing evaluation. Each of the items on the CAPS and CAPS–5 corresponds directly to the *DSM–IV–TR* and *DSM–5* PTSD diagnostic criteria, respectively, and can be anchored to a specific traumatic event. As part of the trauma assessment (Criterion A), the LEC is used to identify traumatic stressors experienced. CAPS items are asked in reference to up to three traumatic stressors. The index trauma can be a single event or several closely related incidents. Both *DSM–IV–TR*- and *DSM–5*-congruent versions of the CAPS provide the clinician with standardized questions to inquire about symptoms, as well as probes to get additional information for diagnostic clarity. In addition to assessing the core PTSD symptoms, questions target the impact of symptoms on social and occupational functioning, improvement in symptoms, overall response validity, overall PTSD severity, and associated features of the disorder (e.g., depersonalization, derealization). Information on these associated features also allows clinicians to properly assess whether an individual meets criteria for the dissociative subtype of PTSD (e.g., Ginzburg et al., 2006; Wolf et al., 2012). The CAPS should be administered by trained clinicians and researchers.

Each of the items on the CAPS for *DSM–IV–TR* requires a clinician rating of symptom frequency and intensity, with each being rated on a 5-point scale (0 = *absent*, 4 = *extreme*). The most frequently used scoring rule is to count a symptom as present if it has a frequency of 1 or more and an intensity of 2 or more. A PTSD diagnosis is made if there is at least 1 B symptom, 3 C symptoms, and 2 D symptoms in addition to meeting the other diagnostic criteria. Severity scores can also be calculated by summing the frequency and intensity ratings for each symptom. Alternative scoring options are described in Weathers, Ruscio, and Keane (1999). The CAPS can be used to evaluate treatment response, with a change in 20 points on the previous version of the CAPS indicated a clinically significant change (Monson et al., 2008). The severity score and the diagnostic outcome can also be used to inform treatment decisions. In addition to accurately reflecting the PTSD diagnostic criteria changes in *DSM–5*, other explicit goals for the CAPS–5 revision were to (a) reduce administration time, (b) facilitate administration and scoring, and (c) adopt a single 5-point rating scale for PTSD symptom severity (0 = *absent*, 4 = *extreme*). Similar to the CAPS for *DSM–IV–TR*, however, a symptom is counted as present if it has a severity rating of 2 (moderate/threshold) or more.

Several other interview instruments can be used to assess PTSD and related psychopathology. The PTSD Symptom Scale Interview (PSS–I; Foa, Riggs, Dancu, & Rothbaum, 1993) is a 17-item *DSM–IV–TR*-correspondent semistructured interview that assesses severity of PTSD related to a single traumatic event. The PSS–I uses single items without probes or follow-up questions. Questions are anchored to the past 2 weeks, and the interviewer scores each item to reflect both frequency and severity on a Likert scale (0 = *not at all*, to 3 = *5 or more times per week/very much*). The Structured Interview for PTSD (SI–PTSD; Davidson, Kudler, & Smith, 1990) is another option for clinicians to use for the assessment and diagnosis of PTSD. It is a brief interview that assesses *DSM*-correspondent PTSD symptoms as well as trauma-related guilt. Each item is rated on severity, which includes both frequency and intensity. Given the diagnostic criterion changes for *DSM–5*, the PSS–I and SI–PTSD will undergo revisions to remain consistent with the updated diagnostic guidelines. Although the *ICD* is currently being revised, to date there are no published *ICD–11* diagnostic measures for PTSD.

ASSESSMENT OF COMORBIDITY AND FUNCTIONAL IMPAIRMENT

PTSD is characterized by high comorbidity with other psychiatric conditions and significant functional impairment (Kessler, Sonnega, Bromet, Hughes, & Nelson, 1995; Kessler, 2000). As a result, conducting a broad-spectrum assessment to assess other disorders is recommended to better inform case conceptualization and treatment planning.

The Structured Clinical Interview for the *DSM–IV–TR* Axis I Disorders (SCID–I; Spitzer et al., 1999) is a semistructured diagnostic interview that assesses all *DSM–IV–TR* Axis I disorders, including PTSD, and averages 90 minutes to complete with psychiatric patients. Using the SCID, clinicians rate the presence or absence of symptoms and other criteria for mental disorders that are of interest and then apply the relevant *DSM–IV–TR* algorithms to determine if the respondent meets criteria for the disorder(s) being assessed. The MINI-International Neuropsychiatric Interview (MINI; Sheehan et al., 1998) is a briefer, structured *DSM–IV–TR* and *ICD–10* correspondent diagnostic interview that covers a range of disorders, including mood, anxiety, and eating disorders, as well as substance use disorders, suicidality, psychotic disorders, and antisocial personality disorder. The MINI was designed for large epidemiological studies and clinical trials to capture routine information and maximize efficiency during medical appointments and takes approximately 15 minutes to administer. Although the SCID–I and MINI have their own PTSD modules, clinicians who want to assess PTSD symptom severity may wish to substitute the CAPS, PSS-I, or another interview instrument that assesses this information. The Anxiety Disorders Interview Schedule for *DSM* (ADIS; Brown, DiNardo, & Barlow, 2004) is another semistructured interview that assesses a range of *DSM* disorders, including, anxiety, mood, somatoform, and substance use disorders. The ADIS can be used to assess current and lifetime diagnoses. Similar to the CAPS and PSS-I, the ADIS provides clinicians with a continuous assessment of symptom severity, which can then be used to determine presence or absence of a disorder.

The Patient Health Questionnaire (PHQ; Spitzer, Kroenke, & Williams, 1999) is a screening and diagnostic self-report measure for a range of disorders that often co-occur with PTSD, including depression, anxiety, and alcohol use. The PHQ can be used to initially assess for additional psychopathology and/or as a means of tracking symptoms change over time.

Additionally, assessing functioning in patients who have experienced trauma provides information about the various domains that are affected by their traumatic event. Currently, clinicians can choose from a number of instruments to assess functioning as part of their assessment battery. In response to many of the limitations of the available self-report instruments (e.g., difficulty in scoring, requiring causal attributions on the part of the respondent), our group has developed a new measure, the Inventory of Psychosocial Functioning (IPF; Rodriguez, Holowka, & Marx, 2012). The IPF assesses impairment within the past 30 days across multiple psychosocial domains of functioning with sufficient breadth and depth without requiring respondents to make attributions regarding the cause of the impairments. Respondents answer each item by using a 7-point scale ranging from 0 (*never*) to 6 (*always*). The IPF yields an overall functional impairment score as well as scores for seven domains: Romantic Relationships, Family Relationships, Work, Friendships and Socializing, Parenting, Academic Pursuits, and Self-Care. Higher scores indicate greater functional impairment.

The World Health Organization Disability Assessment Schedule (WHODAS; Üstün, Kostanjsek, Chatterji, & Rehm, 2010) is another reliable and valid measure that provides information on levels of disability. The WHODAS covers six domains: Cognition (understanding and communication), Mobility (moving and getting around), Self-Care (e.g., hygiene, eating), Getting Along (interacting with others), Life Activities, (e.g., leisure, work), and Participation in Society (engagement in community activities). The WHODAS can be administered as a self-report measure, an interview, or by proxy in which a third party, such as a family member, may provide information on functioning across these domains. The questions are anchored to the past 30 days, and individuals are asked to indicate the level of difficulty by taking into account the way they would typically perform a given activity (including support from an aid). For each item endorsed as *difficult*, individuals are asked to indicated how often the occurred, from 1 = *only one day* to 5 = *every day* (= 30 days). Additionally, individuals are asked to rate degree of interference. A number of studies have used the WHODAS with PTSD samples (e.g., O'Donnell, Creamer, McFarlane, Silove, & Bryant, 2010; Speroff et al., 2012).

CONCLUSION

In this chapter, we briefly reviewed risk factors, diagnostic criteria, and the gold-standard assessment instruments for PTSD and related conditions. Although initial research suggests minimal change in PTSD prevalence rates when using *DSM–5* diagnostic criteria, additional research should examine the impact of *DSM–5*-consistent assessment measures on PTSD prevalence rates. The assessment instruments reviewed in this chapter can guide clinicians with respect to clinical diagnosis as well as treatment planning. Although clinicians are often limited with respect to time with patients, we recommend using a multimethod assessment approach whenever possible to maximize diagnostic accuracy. Using the recommended assessment instruments before, during, and after treatment can provide clinicians with valuable information about patients' progress and inform clinical decisions as part of an ongoing case conceptualization.

REFERENCES

American Psychiatric Association. (2000). *Diagnostic and statistical manual of mental disorders* (4th ed., text rev.). Washington, DC: Author.

American Psychiatric Association. (2013). *Diagnostic and statistical manual of mental disorders* (5th ed.). Arlington, VA: Author.

Andrews, B., Brewin, C. R., Rose, S., & Kirk, M. (2000). Predicting PTSD symptoms in victims of violent crime: The role of shame, anger, and childhood abuse. *Journal of Abnormal Psychology, 109*, 69–73. doi:10.1037/0021-843X.109.1.69

Blake, D. D., Weathers, F. W., Nagy, L. M., Kaloupek, D. G., Gusman, F. D., Charney, D. S., & Keane, T. M. (1995). The development of a clinician-administered PTSD scale. *Journal of Traumatic Stress, 8*, 75–90. doi:10.1002/jts.2490080106

Blanchard, E. B., Hickling, E. J., Taylor, A. E., & Loos, W. (1995). Psychiatric morbidity associated with motor vehicle accidents. *Journal of Nervous and Mental Disease, 183*, 495–504. doi:10.1097/00005053-199508000-00001

Bovin, M. J., & Marx, B. P. (2011). The importance of the peritraumatic experience in defining traumatic stress. *Psychological Bulletin, 137*, 47–67. doi:10.1037/a0021353

Bovin, M. J., & Weathers, F. W. (2012). Assessing PTSD Symptoms. In J. G. Beck & D. M. Sloan (Eds.), *The Oxford handbook of traumatic stress disorders* (pp. 235–249). New York, NY: Oxford University Press.

Breslau, N., Davis, G. C., Andreski, P., & Peterson, E. (1991). Traumatic events and posttraumatic stress disorder in an urban population of young adults. *Archives of General Psychiatry, 48*, 216–222. doi:10.1001/archpsyc.1991.01810270028003

Breslau, N., Peterson, E. L., Kessler, R. C., & Schultz, L. R. (1999). Short screening scale for *DSM–IV* posttraumatic stress disorder. *The American Journal of Psychiatry, 156*, 908–911.

Brewin, C. R., Andrews, B., & Valentine, J. D. (2000). Meta-analysis of risk factors for posttraumatic stress disorder in trauma-exposed adults. *Journal of Consulting and Clinical Psychology, 68*, 748–766. doi:10.1037/0022-006X.68.5.748

Bromet, E., Sonnega, A., & Kessler, R. C. (1998). Risk factors for *DSM–III–R* posttraumatic stress disorder: Findings from the National Comorbidity Survey. *American Journal of Epidemiology, 147*, 353–361. doi:10.1093/oxfordjournals.aje.a009457

Brown, T. A., DiNardo, P., & Barlow, D. H. (2004). *Anxiety Disorders Interview Schedule (ADIS–IV)*. Boulder, CO: Graywind.

Calhoun, P. S., Hertzberg, J. S., Kirby, A. C., Dennis, M. F., Hair, L. P., Dedert, E. A., & Beckham, J. C. (2012). The effect of draft *DSM–V* criteria on posttraumatic stress disorder prevalence. *Depression and Anxiety, 29*, 1032–1042. doi:10.1002/da.22012

Connor, K. M., & Davidson, J. R. (2001). SPRINT: A brief global assessment of post-traumatic stress disorder. *International Clinical Psychopharmacology, 16*, 279–284. doi:10.1097/00004850-200109000-00005

Cornelis, M. C., Nugent, N. R., Amstadter, A. B., & Koenen, K. C. (2010). Genetics of post-traumatic stress disorder: Review and recommendations for genome-wide association studies. *Current Psychiatry Reports, 12*, 313–326. doi:10.1007/s11920-010-0126-6

Davidson, J. R. T., Book, S. W., Colket, J. T., Tupler, L. A., Roth, S., David, D., ... Feldman, M. (1997). Assessment of a new self-rating scale for post-traumatic stress disorder. *Psychological Medicine, 27*, 153–160. doi:10.1017/S0033291796004229

Davidson, J. R. T., Kudler, H. S., & Smith, R. D. (1990). Assessment and pharmacotherapy of posttraumatic stress disorder. In J. E. L. Giller (Ed.), *Biological assessment and treatment of posttraumatic stress disorder* (pp. 205–221). Washington, DC: American Psychiatric Press.

Delahanty, D. L., Raimonde, A. J., Spoonster, E., & Cullado, M. (2003). Injury severity, prior trauma history, urinary cortisol levels and acute PTSD in motor vehicle accident victims. *Journal of Anxiety Disorders, 17,* 149–164. doi:10.1016/S0887-6185(02)00185-8

Derogatis, L. R. (1994). *Symptom Checklist—90* (rev. ed.). Minneapolis, MN: Pearson Assessments.

Foa, E. B., Cashman, L., Jaycox, L., & Perry, K. (1997). The validation of a self-report measure of PTSD: The Posttraumatic Diagnostic Scale. *Psychological Assessment, 9,* 445–451. doi:10.1037/1040-3590.9.4.445

Foa, E. B., Riggs, D. S., Dancu, C. V., & Rothbaum, B. O. (1993). Reliability and validity of a brief instrument for assessing post-traumatic stress disorder. *Journal of Traumatic Stress, 6,* 459–473. doi:10.1002/jts.2490060405

Ginzburg, K., Koopman, C., Butler, L. D., Palesh, O., Kraemer, H. C., Classen, C. C., & Spiegel, D. (2006). Evidence for a dissociative subtype of post-traumatic stress disorder among help-seeking childhood sexual abuse survivors. *Journal of Trauma & Dissociation, 7,* 7–27. doi:10.1300/J229v07n02_02

Green, B. (1996). Trauma History Questionnaire. In B. H. Stamm (Ed.), *Measurement of stress, trauma, and adaptation* (pp. 366–369). Lutherville, MD: Sidran Press.

Hoge, C. W., Castro, C. A., Messer, S. C., McGurk, D., Cotting, D. I., & Koffman, R. L. (2004). Combat duty in Iraq and Afghanistan, mental health problems, and barriers to care. *The New England Journal of Medicine, 351,* 13–22. doi:10.1056/NEJMoa040603

Keane, T. M., Caddell, J. M., & Taylor, K. L. (1988). Mississippi Scale for Combat-Related Posttraumatic Stress Disorder: Three studies in reliability and validity. *Journal of Consulting and Clinical Psychology, 56,* 85–90. doi:10.1037/0022-006X.56.1.85

Keane, T. M., Malloy, P. F., & Fairbanks, J. A. (1984). Empirical development of an MMPI subscale for the assessment of combat-related posttraumatic stress disorder. *Journal of Consulting and Clinical Psychology, 52,* 888–891. doi:10.1037/0022-006X.52.5.888

Kessler, R. C. (2000). Posttraumatic stress disorder: The burden to the individual and to society. *Journal of Clinical Psychiatry, 61*(Suppl. 5), 4–12.

Kessler, R. C., Sonnega, A., Bromet, E., Hughes, M., & Nelson, C. B. (1995). Posttraumatic stress disorder in the National Comorbidity Survey. *Archives of General Psychiatry, 52,* 1048–1060. doi:10.1001/archpsyc.1995.03950240066012

King, D. W., King, L. A., Foy, D. W., & Gudanowski, D. M. (1996). Prewar factors in combat-related posttraumatic stress disorder: Structural equation modeling with a national sample of female and male Vietnam veterans. *Journal of Consulting and Clinical Psychology*, 64, 520–531. doi:10.1037/0022-006X. 64.3.520

King, D. W., King, L. A., Gudanowski, D. M., & Vreven, D. L. (1995). Alternative representations of war zone stressors: Relationships to posttraumatic stress disorder in male and female Vietnam veterans. *Journal of Abnormal Psychology*, 104, 184–195. doi:10.1037/0021-843X.104.1.184

King, L. A., King, D. W., Salgado, D. M., & Shalev, A. Y. (2003). Contemporary longitudinal methods for the study of trauma and posttraumatic stress disorder. *CNS Spectrums*, 8, 686–692.

Krinsley, K. E., Gallagher, J. G., Weathers, F. W., Kaloupek, D. G., & Vielhauer, M. (1997). *Reliability and validity of the Evaluation of Lifetime Stressors questionnaire*. Unpublished manuscript.

Kubany, E. S., Haynes, S. N., Leisen, M. B., Owens, J. A., Kaplan, A. S., Watson, S. B., & Burns, K. (2000). Development and preliminary validation of a brief broad-spectrum measure of trauma exposure: The Traumatic Life Events Questionnaire. *Psychological Assessment*, 12, 210–224. doi:10.1037/1040-3590. 12.2.210

Maercker, A., Brewin, C. R., Bryant, R. A., Cloitre, M., Ommeren, M., Jones, L. M., . . . Reed, G. M. (2013). Diagnosis and classification of disorders specifically associated with stress: Proposals for ICD–11. *World Psychiatry*, 12, 198–206. doi:10.1002/wps.20057

McDonald, S. D., & Calhoun, P. S. (2010). The diagnostic accuracy of the PTSD checklist: A critical review. *Clinical Psychology Review*, 30, 976–987. doi:10.1016/j.cpr.2010.06.012

Meltzer-Brody, S., Churchill, E., & Davidson, J. R. (1999). Derivation of the SPAN, a brief diagnostic screening test for post-traumatic stress disorder. *Psychiatry Research*, 88, 63–70. doi:10.1016/S0165-1781(99)00070-0

Miller, M. W., Wolf, E. J., Kilpatrick, D., Resnick, H., Marx, B. P., Holowka, D. W., . . . Friedman, M. J. (2013). The prevalence and latent structure of proposed *DSM–5* posttraumatic stress disorder symptoms in U.S. national and veteran samples. *Psychological Trauma: Theory, Research, Practice, and Policy*, 5, 501–512. doi:10.1037/a0029730

Monson, C. M., Gradus, J. L., Young-Xu, Y., Schnurr, P. P., Price, J. L., & Schumm, J. A. (2008). Change in posttraumatic stress disorder symptoms: Do clinicians and patients agree? *Psychological Assessment*, 20, 131–138. doi:10.1037/1040-3590.20.2.131

Nishith, P., Mechanic, M. B., & Resick, P. A. (2000). Prior interpersonal trauma: The contribution to current PTSD symptoms in female rape victims. *Journal of Abnormal Psychology, 109,* 20–25. doi:10.1037/0021-843X.109.1.20

O'Donnell, M. L., Creamer, M. C., McFarlane, A. C., Silove, D., & Bryant, R. A. (2010). Does access to compensation have an impact on recovery outcomes after injury? *The Medical Journal of Australia, 192,* 328–333.

Ozer, E. J., Best, S. R., Lipsey, T. L., & Weiss, D. S. (2003). Predictors of posttraumatic stress disorder and symptoms in adults: A meta-analysis. *Psychological Bulletin, 129,* 52–73. doi:10.1037/0033-2909.129.1.52

Prins, A., Ouimette, P., Kimerling, R., Cameron, R. P., Hugelshofer, D. S., Shaw-Hegwer, J., . . . Sheikh, J. I. (2004). The primary care PTSD screen (PC-PTSD): Development and operating characteristics. *Primary Care Psychiatry, 9,* 9–14. doi:10.1185/135525703125002360

Rodriguez, P., Holowka, D. W., & Marx, B. P. (2012). Assessment of posttraumatic stress disorder-related functional impairment: A review. *Journal of Rehabilitation Research and Development, 49,* 649–665. doi:10.1682/JRRD.2011.09.0162

Sheehan, D. V., Lecrubier, Y., Sheehan, K. H., Amorim, P., Janavs, J., Weiller, E., . . . Dunbar, G. C. (1998). The Mini-International Neuropsychiatric Interview (MINI): The development and validation of a structured diagnostic psychiatric interview for *DSM–IV* and *ICD-10. Journal of Clinical Psychiatry, 59,* 22–33.

Speroff, T., Sinnott, P. L., Marx, B., Owen, R. R., Jackson, J. C., Greevy, R., . . . Friedman, M. J. (2012). Impact of evidence-based standardized assessment on the disability clinical interview for diagnosis of service-connected PTSD: A cluster-randomized trial. *Journal of Traumatic Stress, 25,* 607–615. doi:10.1002/jts.21759

Spitzer, R. L., Kroenke, K., & Williams, J. B. W. (1999). Validation and utility of a self-report version of PRIME-MD. *JAMA, 282,* 1737–1744. doi:10.1001/jama.282.18.1737

Üstün, T. B., Kostanjsek, N., Chatterji, S., & Rehm, J. (Eds.). (2010). *Measuring health and disability: Manual for WHO Disability Assessment Schedule (WHODAS 2.0).* Geneva, Switzerland: World Health Organization.

Vogt, D., Smith, B. N., King, D. W., & King, L. A. (2012). *Manual for the Deployment Risk and Resilience Inventory—2 (DRRI–2): A collection of measures for studying deployment-related experiences of military veterans.* Boston, MA: National Center for PTSD.

Vrana, S., & Lauterbach, D. (1994). Prevalence of traumatic events and posttraumatic psychological symptoms in a nonclinical sample of college students. *Journal of Traumatic Stress, 7,* 289–302. doi:10.1002/jts.2490070209

Weathers, F., Blake, D. D., Schnurr, P. P., Kaloupek, D. G., Marx, B. P., & Keane, T. M. (2012). *Clinician Administered PTSD Scale for DSM–5*. Unpublished manuscript.

Weathers, F., Litz, B., Herman, D., Huska, J., & Keane, T. M. (1993, October). *The PTSD Checklist (PCL): Reliability, validity, and diagnostic utility*. Paper presented at the Annual Convention of the International Society for Traumatic Stress Studies, San Antonio, TX.

Weathers, F., Litz, B., Keane, T. M., Palmieri, P. P., Marx, B. P., & Schnurr, P. P. (2010). *PTSD Checklist for DSM–5*. Unpublished manuscript.

Weathers, F. W., Keane, T. M., & Davidson, J. R. (2001). Clinician-administered PTSD scale: A review of the first ten years of research. *Depression and Anxiety, 13*, 132–156. doi:10.1002/da.1029

Weathers, F. W., Keane, T. M., & Foa, E. B. (2009). Assessment and diagnosis of adults. In E. B. Foa, T. M. Keane, M. J. Friedman, & J. A. Cohen (Eds.), *Effective treatments for PTSD: Practice guidelines from the international society for traumatic stress studies* (pp. 23–61). New York, NY: Guilford Press.

Weathers, F. W., Ruscio, A. M., & Keane, T. M. (1999). Psychometric properties of nine scoring rules for the Clinician-Administered Posttraumatic Stress Disorder Scale. *Psychological Assessment, 11*, 124–133. doi:10.1037/1040-3590.11.2.124

Weiss, D. S., & Marmar, C. R. (1996). The Impact of Event Scale—Revised. In J. Wilson & T. M. Keane (Eds.), *Assessing psychological trauma and PTSD* (pp. 399–411). New York, NY: Guilford Press.

Wilkins, K. C., Lang, A. J., & Norman, S. B. (2011). Synthesis of the psychometric properties of the PTSD Checklist (PCL) military, civilian, and specific versions. *Depression and Anxiety, 28*, 596–606. doi:10.1002/da.20837

Wolf, E. J., Miller, M. W., Reardon, A. F., Ryabchenko, K. A., Castillo, D., & Freund, R. (2012). A latent class analysis of dissociation and PTSD: Evidence for a dissociative subtype. *Archives of General Psychiatry, 69*, 698–705. doi:10.1001/archgenpsychiatry.2011.1574

TWO

PHARMACOLOGICAL AND PSYCHOTHERAPEUTIC APPROACHES

4

Antidepressant Strategies in the Management of PTSD

Nancy C. Bernardy and Matthew J. Friedman

This chapter seeks to provide an overview of the research on the use of antidepressants in patients with a diagnosis of posttraumatic stress disorder (PTSD). It reviews newer medication strategies that build on recent research based on our improved understanding of the neurobiology of PTSD, including the use of sympatholytics, and offers information on novel alternative treatment recommendations to clinicians to address the complex array of symptoms in those individuals who have a PTSD diagnosis.

RESEARCH ON MEDICATION USE FOR PTSD TREATMENT

The first randomized clinical trials (RCTs) testing effective medications for PTSD focused on antidepressants. Around 1990, a few reports on small, single-site RCTs had been published indicating the effectiveness of the

http://dx.doi.org/10.1037/14522-005
A Practical Guide to PTSD Treatment: Pharmacological and Psychotherapeutic Approaches,
N. C. Bernardy and M. J. Friedman (Editors)
Copyright © 2015 by the American Psychological Association. All rights reserved.

tricyclic antidepressants (TCAs) imipramine and amitriptyline and the monoamine oxidase inhibitor (MAOI) phenelzine (Friedman, Davidson, & Stein, 2009). Since 2000, however, spurred greatly by industry-sponsored trials of selective serotonin reuptake inhibitors (SSRIs), significant progress has been made in the pharmacotherapy of PTSD, due primarily to the recognition of the overlap of PTSD symptoms with those of depression and many anxiety disorders. The bulk of research through industry-sponsored multisite RCTs has examined SSRIs (especially sertraline, paroxetine, and fluoxetine) with more than 3,000 patients and has found them to be effective in treating PTSD (Friedman et al., 2009). On the basis of such trials (Brady et al., 2000; Davidson et al., 2001; Marshall, Beebe, Oldham, & Zaninelli, 2001; Tucker et al., 2001), paroxetine and sertraline have U.S. Food and Drug Administration (FDA) approval for PTSD, are generally well tolerated, and are recommended as first-line agents in several treatment guidelines (Forbes et al., 2010). However, clinicians have received mixed messages on the efficacy of SSRIs for PTSD, and this has been particularly true in veteran populations. The prestigious Institute of Medicine (IOM) report, issued in 2007 to assess the evidence on PTSD treatment options, concluded that for all drug classes reviewed, the research evidence was inadequate to determine efficacy in the management of PTSD. The World Health Organization (WHO; 2013) recently published its new guidelines on the treatment of traumatic stress, which followed the United Kingdom's National Institute for Clinical Excellence (NICE, 2005) guidelines in recommending antidepressants for adults with PTSD when psychological treatments are not available or have not been effective, as well as for people who have concurrent moderate to severe depression (Tol, Barbui, & van Ommeren, 2013). In contrast, the latest Agency for Healthcare Research and Quality (AHRQ; 2013) report shows reasonably good effect sizes for paroxetine and the selective norepinephrine/serotonin reuptake inhibitor (SNRI) venlafaxine, but less strong effects for other SSRIs and negative effects for citalopram. Thus, progress has been made, but the findings are still mixed.

ANTIDEPRESSANTS USED IN TREATING PTSD

FDA approval for sertraline and paroxetine was based on evidence from RCTs with hundreds of participants demonstrating significant reductions in PTSD symptoms compared with placebo as well as remission in 30% of study participants (Brady et al., 2000; Davidson et al., 2001; Marshall et al., 2001; Tucker et al., 2001). A significant open-label study soon followed showing that when sertraline treatment was extended for a longer period of time, from 12 to 36 weeks, remission rates increased from 30% to 55% (Londborg et al., 2001). Additional research has examined relapse and has found that discontinuation of sertraline and fluoxetine is associated with clinical relapse and a return of PTSD symptoms (Davidson, Baldwin, et al., 2006; Davidson et al., 2001; Marshall et al., 2007; Martenyi, Brown, Zhang, Koke, & Prakash, 2002; Rapaport, Endicott, & Clary, 2002).

SSRIs and SNRIs

Further RCTs with SSRIs soon followed, with similar efficacious results compared with placebo; these studies are evaluated in several recent reviews (Friedman, 2013; Friedman & Davidson, 2014; Ipser, Seedat, & Stein, 2006; Stein, Ipser, & Seedat, 2006). Most clinical practice guidelines for PTSD recognize this body of work and recommend SSRIs and the SNRI venlafaxine as first-line monotherapy for PTSD (Forbes et al., 2010; U.S. Department of Veterans Affairs & Department of Defense [VA/DoD], 2010). The two guidelines that did not follow with this recommendation are the previously mentioned IOM (2007) report and the United Kingdom's NICE (2005) guidelines, the basis of the recent WHO (2013) report. The stringent criteria of the IOM report excluded several studies that supported the recommendation of SSRIs in other guidelines, whereas NICE did just the opposite and included unpublished studies and did not consider results with an effect size under 0.5 as positive (Friedman, 2013; Friedman & Davidson, 2014).

A number of trials, however, have failed to show any differences between SSRIs and placebo, and these have contributed to confusion about the use of SSRIs for PTSD (Brady et al., 2005; Davidson, Rothbaum, et al., 2006; Friedman, Marmar, Baker, Sikes, & Farfel, 2007; Martenyi, Brown, & Caldwell, 2007; Shalev et al., 2012; Tucker et al., 2003; Zohar et al., 2002). The mixed results may be due to unexpectedly strong placebo responses and the chronicity of some patient cohorts (Friedman & Davidson, 2014).

Large multicenter trials later turned to newer antidepressants, termed SNRIs, that block reuptake not only of serotonin but also of norepinephrine. Two large multicenter trials of venlafaxine-XR, one of which was 12 weeks in duration (Davidson, Rothbaum, et al., 2006; Tucker et al., 2001) and the other 6 months in duration (Davidson, Baldwin, et al., 2006), have shown superiority relative to placebo. Interesting results have been noted in the venlafaxine trials, including significant improvements on measures of resilience, ability to deal with daily stress, and anger and aggression (Davidson et al., 2012; Stein et al., 2009). Similar to findings in SSRIs, the 6-month trial noted that a substantial percentage of patients achieved remission only after several months of treatment (Davidson, Rothbaum, et al., 2006; Marshall et al., 2001).

Despite the conflicting recommendations, the use of SSRIs as a first-line treatment for PTSD has increased. Research that examined prescribing patterns in veterans with a diagnosis of PTSD receiving treatment in Veterans Affairs facilities found that over a 10-year period from 1999 to 2009, prescribing frequency of SSRIs increased from 49.7% to 59% (Bernardy, Lund, Alexander, & Friedman, 2012). Overall, this widespread increase in SSRI use among military veterans is consistent with guideline-concordant care and has been noted by others (Mohamed & Rosenheck, 2008). Clearly prescribing clinicians believe that veterans benefit from these medications. It has been suggested that the widespread SSRI treatment is especially effective for PTSD symptoms such as irritability, anger, depression, and anxiety (Shiromani, Keane, & LeDoux, 2012); however, other symptoms within the fourth edition (text revision) of the *Diagnostic and Statistical Manual of Mental Disorders* (*DSM–IV–TR;* American Psychiatric Association, 2000) intrusion, avoidance, and numbing clusters also appear responsive to SSRI pharmacotherapy (Friedman, 2013).

Mirtazapine, Nefazodone, and Trazodone

Mirtazapine, another antidepressant that enhances serotonergic (5-HT) activity and also has action at presynaptic alpha-2 adrenergic receptors, has proven efficacious as monotherapy for PTSD. It is recommended as a second-line agent (Forbes et al., 2010; Friedman et al., 2009; Londborg et al., 2001; Tol et al., 2013). The sexual side effects of mirtazapine are often lower than the other SSRIs, making it an effective alternative. Nefazodone and trazodone are two antidepressants that have also been studied in PTSD. Nefazodone acts by blocking presynaptic 5-HT reuptake while antagonizing postsynaptic $5-HT_2$ receptors; it has been shown to be as effective as sertraline in several RCTs (Forbes et al., 2010; VA/DoD, 2010). Despite these positive findings, particularly on the difficult-to-target hyperarousal symptoms, nefazodone has received a black box warning for hepatotoxicity. It has been mostly withdrawn from the U.S. market (as Desyrel), although generic nefazodone is still available (it should only be prescribed for patients who do not respond to SSRIs, and liver enzymes must be closely monitored; Friedman & Davidson, 2014). Trazodone, which has similar actions as nefazodone, has limited efficacy and is not recommended as monotherapy for PTSD (VA/DoD, 2010). Trazodone does have effective sedating actions and is thus often used at low doses adjunctively with SSRIs to promote sleep as well as for insomnia due to other causes (Friedman, Davidson, & Stein, 2009).

TCAs and MAOIs

TCAs and MAOIs are also recommended as second-line agents (Forbes et al., 2010; VA/DoD, 2010). The MAOI phenelzine has shown some benefit in an RCT with Vietnam combat veterans, reducing reexperiencing and arousal symptoms (Kosten, Frank, Dan, McDougle, & Giller, 1991). However, despite their recommendation as second-line monotherapies for PTSD, neither TCAs nor MAOIs are frequently used or studied today; compared with SNRIs, they have riskier side-effect profiles and much less research support (Friedman & Davidson, 2014). MAOIs and TCAs do remain important options for PTSD patients, particularly for those with major depressive symptoms. A recent study indicated that the TCA desipramine may be a good choice for PTSD patients with co-occurring substance use disorder (Petrakis et al., 2012).

Nonserotonergic Agents

With a greater understanding of the psychobiology of PTSD, recent work has shifted its focus from serotonergic agents. A promising area of research has investigated the use of a sympatholytic, prazosin, an alpha-1-adrenergic postsynaptic antagonist, as an effective treatment for PTSD-related nightmares. Prazosin's antagonism of central nervous system adrenergic activity is strongly associated with reduction of PTSD-related nightmares. In four relatively small studies (Raskind et al., 2000, 2002, 2003; Taylor & Raskind, 2002) evening doses of prazosin significantly reduced traumatic nightmares and had mixed results regarding amelioration of the full PTSD syndrome. A recent RCT with military personnel had positive results on both daytime and sleep-associated symptoms in which the medication was administered twice daily, in morning and evening doses (Raskind et al., 2013). This work noted improvements in total PTSD symptom severity, especially with respect to arousal symptoms, as well as improvements in trauma-related nightmares, sleep quality, and global functioning. Increased use of prazosin nationally among veterans with PTSD has been recently observed (Bernardy et al., 2012). Interesting areas of future research include combinations of effective psychotherapy treatments for PTSD with prazosin.

In contrast to the exciting findings regarding prazosin, early reports of beneficial effects of a beta-adrenergic antagonist, propranolol, have not led to RCTs testing its efficacy for PTSD. Instead, propranolol has been mostly studied as a potential acute posttraumatic pharmacological intervention to prevent the development of PTSD (see Friedman &

Davidson, 2014). However, this line of work has not shown that propranolol is an effective prophylactic agent compared with placebo, so it is not recommended as an acute intervention in the guidelines (VA/DoD, 2010). Recent research with propranolol has tested the possibility that it might ameliorate chronic PTSD by disrupting the reconsolidation of traumatic memories (Poundja, Sanche, Tremblay, & Brunet, 2012). This theoretically driven approach is exciting and awaits the necessary RCT evaluation.

Similarly, alpha-2 adrenergic agonists would be expected to be effective in treating PTSD, given the antagonism of presynaptic norepinephrine release. The limited (non-RCT) work examining the efficacy of clonidine in PTSD is generally favorable (Kinzie, 2004; Kolb, Burris, & Griffiths, 1984). However, two RCTs with guanfacine in veterans with PTSD have been negative (Friedman & Davidson, 2014).

Anticonvulsant agents that block sensitization and kindling have been tested in small to medium-size trials with generally disappointing results. Negative or equivocal findings have resulted from RCTs with valproate (Davis et al., 2008). Clinical trials with lamotrigine and tiagabine have had similarly disappointing findings (Friedman & Davidson, 2014).

Topiramate, however, has shown the greatest promise of all the anticonvulsant agents. A recent meta-analysis by the AHRQ (2013) concluded that it was at least as effective as paroxetine and venlafaxine. Topiramate has been studied in five double-blind, placebo-controlled trials with mixed results. Exceptional benefit in a group of treatment-resistant patients was noted using topiramate as an augmentation strategy to antidepressants (Akuchekian & Amanat, 2004). However, another study found no overall benefit and suffered from high dropout rates due to side effects from the drug (Lindley et al., 2007). Three monotherapy trials have provided modest but inconsistent results (Petty, Fieve, Capece, & Davis, 2005; Tucker et al., 2007; Yeh et al., 2011). The positive recommendation of topiramate by the AHRQ should be considered in the context of all topiramate trials in PTSD, some of which were omitted in their analysis. Nonetheless, topiramate shows encouraging evidence of efficacy and may be useful in PTSD in patients with the common co-occurring alcohol use disorder or to augment partial responders to SSRIs.

The data regarding the use of benzodiazepines in PTSD are presented in Chapter 5 of this volume. In short, there is no evidence for the efficacy of benzodiazepines and considerable evidence that they pose significant clinical risks. Given such an unfavorable risk–benefit ratio, they are not recommended for treatment of PTSD. An interesting area of research is the positive study of eszopiclone, a nonbenzodiazepine gamma-aminobutyric acid (GABA)-A receptor agonist indicated for the treatment of sleep onset and maintenance insomnia. In this small study of 24 patients with PTSD, 3 weeks of eszopiclone was associated with significantly greater improvement than placebo on PTSD symptom measures as well as on measures of sleep (Pollack et al., 2011). This study provided preliminary evidence that the use of eszopiclone to manage PTSD is associated with short-term improvement in overall symptom severity as well as associated sleep disturbance. Continued work with this agent will provide a clearer picture of its role in the treatment of PTSD. It is interesting that work with a similar agent, zolpidem, has not shown efficacy in the management of PTSD (Abramowitz, Barak, Ben-Avi, & Nobler, 2008) and that new concerns about safety issues with this nonbenzodiazepine hypnotic continue to be noted (Gunja, 2013).

Atypical antipsychotic agents are not recommended in the management of PTSD. Neither conventional nor atypical antipsychotics are recommended as monotherapy for PTSD (for a review, see Chapter 6, this volume).

New research is being conducted with medications that might be expected to target the specific pathophysiology of PTSD. This is different from most previous research, which has tested medications previously developed for treatment of other disorders, such as depression, anxiety disorders, cardiovascular diseases, epilepsy, or psychosis. Such medications might target adrenergic, hypothalamic–pituitary–adrenocortical, glutamatergic, GABA-ergic, inflammatory, or other mechanisms that mediate the human stress response and that are altered among patients with PTSD (see Chapter 1, this volume). For example, a small RCT with chronic PTSD patients observed that hydrocortisone might inhibit reconsolidation of traumatic memories and thus decrease PTSD symptoms (Suris et al.,

2010). Other work involves the use of agents that act on endocannabinoids, oxytocin, neurokinin/substance P, and dopamine (Dunlop, Mansson, & Gerardi, 2012).

CONCLUSION

Antidepressants, especially SNRIs, are recommended as a first-line treatment for PTSD. Full remission is generally achieved in 30% of patients, and clinical improvement is usually noted in an additional 50%. Although at present it appears that cognitive behavior therapy (CBT) may be more effective, an initial trial with pharmacotherapy has much to recommend it because of widespread availability of prescribing clinicians (both psychiatrists and primary care providers). In contrast, there are relatively few CBT therapists qualified to deliver evidence-based CBT, especially outside of the VA Healthcare System and especially in rural areas. Furthermore, as more screening for PTSD is instituted in primary care settings, it is important that primary care providers have an effective therapeutic option, especially for patients who are unwilling to seek treatment in a mental health clinic.

The major focus for clinical pharmacotherapy trials in PTSD has been with serotonergic agents, primarily SSRIs and more recently SNRIs. Most of these clinical trials have been conducted with middle-aged White women who had been sexually assaulted. Although questions have been raised after failed antidepressant strategies, it appears unlikely that combat-related PTSD among men is less responsive than sexual trauma among women to SNRI treatment. It is more likely that negative results among veterans are due to chronicity rather than gender or the specific nature of the trauma (Friedman & Davidson, 2014). Interpretation of results from negative antidepressant trials is also complicated because of unusually high placebo response rates (which would obscure any medication response) and the inadequate data on therapeutic doses and blood levels. Increasing antidepressant dosages to the maximal recommended dose is often needed. Further work is needed examining those patients who fail to respond to first- or second-level interactions. Even when remission from

PTSD is not achieved, recommended first-line pharmacotherapies often reduce irritability, low anger threshold, and depression; such a clinical response can have a large impact on quality of life, even if PTSD persists.

In summary, investigators are making considerable progress in moving forward with recommended interventions for PTSD. Different phenotypes of PTSD (e.g., anxious, depressive, externalizing, dissociative) now acknowledged by the new *DSM–5* criteria (American Psychiatric Association, 2013; Friedman, in press) might be best addressed by different pharmacotherapies. Furthermore, clinicians should determine whether patients who have "failed" previous pharmacological treatments were compliant or received an adequate trial. It may be the case that another SNRI should be prescribed to ensure that the patient has had an adequate therapeutic trial before concluding that he or she is unresponsive to medication. We also look forward to the future availability of effective medications that have been developed specifically to treat the unique pathophysiology of PTSD. However, it is critical that patients and their treating clinicians recognize that at this time, trauma-focused psychotherapies are the first-line recommended treatments to address PTSD. Pharmacotherapy may play an important role, but there are unanswered questions about the length of time patients may need to remain on medications, withdrawal syndromes, and the medications' efficacy for treating the overall disorder. It is important to note that the interactions between pharmacotherapy and psychotherapy need to be examined in well-designed studies. At a time when patient-centered care is an increased focus of the health care system in general, we need to teach providers how to have informed conversations with their patients about the best course of treatment to manage PTSD and then be able to have referral sources to meet those choices.

REFERENCES

Abramowitz, E. G., Barak, Y., Ben-Avi, I., & Nobler, H. Y. (2008). Hypnotherapy in the treatment of chronic combat-related PTSD patients suffering from insomnia: A randomized, zolpidem-controlled clinical trial. *International Journal of Clinical and Experimental Hypnosis, 56,* 270–280. doi:10.1080/00207140802039672

Agency for Healthcare Research and Quality. (2013). *Interventions for the prevention of posttraumatic stress disorder (PTSD) in adults after exposure to psychological trauma*. Rockville, MD: Author. Retrieved from http://www.effectivehealthcare.ahrq.gov

Akuchekian, S., & Amanat, S. (2004). The comparison of topiramate and placebo in the treatment of posttraumatic stress disorder: A randomized, double-blind study. *Journal of Research in Medical Sciences, 9*, 240–244.

American Psychiatric Association. (2000). *Diagnostic and statistical manual of mental disorders* (4th ed., text rev.). Washington, DC: Author.

American Psychiatric Association. (2013). *Diagnostic and statistical manual of mental disorders* (5th ed.). Washington, DC: Author.

Bernardy, N. C., Lund, B. C., Alexander, B., & Friedman, M. J. (2012). Prescribing trends in veterans with posttraumatic stress disorder. *Journal of Clinical Psychiatry, 73*, 297–303. doi:10.4088/JCP.11m07311

Brady, K., Pearlstein, T., Asnis, G. M., Baker, D., Rothbaum, B., Sikes, C. R., & Farfel, G. M. (2000). Efficacy and safety of sertraline treatment of posttraumatic stress disorder: A randomized controlled trial. *JAMA, 283*, 1837–1844. doi:10.1001/jama.283.14.1837

Brady, K. T., Sonne, S., Anton, R. F., Randall, C. L., Back, S. E., & Simpson, K. (2005). Sertraline in the treatment of co-occurring alcohol dependence and posttraumatic stress disorder. *Alcoholism: Clinical and Experimental Research, 29*, 395–401. doi:10.1097/01.ALC.0000156129.98265.57

Davidson, J., Baldwin, D. V., Stein, D. J., Kuper, E., Benattia, I., Ahmed, S., . . . Musgnung, J. (2006). Treatment of posttraumatic stress disorder with venlafaxine extended release: A 6-month randomized controlled trial. *Archives of General Psychiatry, 63*, 1158–1165. doi:10.1001/archpsyc.63.10.1158

Davidson, J., Pearlstein, T., Londborg, P., Brady, K. T., Rothbaum, B., Bell, J., . . . Farfel, G. (2001). Efficacy of sertraline in preventing relapse of posttraumatic stress disorder: Results of a 28-week double-blind, placebo-controlled study. *The American Journal of Psychiatry, 158*, 1974–1981. doi:10.1176/appi.ajp.158.12.1974

Davidson, J., Rothbaum, B. O., Tucker, P., Asnis, G., Benattia, I., & Musgnung, J. J. (2006). Venlafaxine extended release in posttraumatic stress disorder: A sertraline- and placebo-controlled study [corrected in *Journal of Clinical Psychopharmacology, 26*, 473; dosage error in article text]. *Journal of Clinical Psychopharmacology, 26*, 259–267. doi:10.1097/01.jcp.0000222514.71390.c1

Davidson, J., Stein, D. J., Rothbaum, B. O., Pedersen, R., Szumski, A., & Baldwin, D. S. (2012). Resilience as a predictor of treatment response in patients with posttraumatic stress disorder treated with venlafaxine extended release or placebo. *Journal of Psychopharmacology, 26,* 778–783. doi:10.1177/026988 1111413821

Davis, L. L., Davidson, J. R. T., Ward, L. C., Bartolucci, A. A., Bowden, C., & Petty, F. (2008). Divalproex in the treatment of posttraumatic stress disorder: A randomized double-blind, placebo-controlled trial in a veteran population. *Journal of Clinical Psychopharmacology, 28,* 84–88. doi:10.1097/JCP.0b013e318160f83b

Dunlop, B. W., Mansson, E., & Gerardi, M. (2012). Pharmacological innovations for posttraumatic stress disorder and medication-enhanced psychotherapy. *Current Pharmaceutical Design, 18,* 5645–5658. doi:10.2174/138161212803530899

Forbes, D., Creamer, M. C., Bisson, J. I., Cohen, J. A., Crow, B. E., Foa, E. B., . . . Ursano, R. J. (2010). A guide to guidelines for the treatment of PTSD and related conditions. *Journal of Traumatic Stress, 23,* 537–552. doi:10.1002/jts.20565

Friedman, M. J. (2013, July 1). PTSD: Pharmacotherapeutic approaches. *Focus Psychiatry Online,* 315–320.

Friedman, M. J. (in press). Deconstructing PTSD. In E. J. Bromet (Ed.), *Long-term outcomes in psychopathology research: Rethinking the scientific agenda.* New York, NY: Oxford University Press.

Friedman, M. J., & Davidson, J. R. T. (2014). Pharmacotherapy for PTSD. In M. J. Friedman, T. M. Keane, & P. A. Resick (Eds.), *Handbook of PTSD: Science and practice* (2nd ed., pp. 482–501). New York, NY: Guilford Press.

Friedman, M. J., Davidson, J. R. T., & Stein, D. J. (2009). Psychopharmacotherapy for adults. In E. B. Foa, T. M. Keane, M. J. Friedman, & J. A. Cohen (Eds.), *Effective treatments for PTSD: Practice guidelines from the International Society for Traumatic Stress Studies* (2nd ed., pp. 245–268). New York, NY: Guilford Press.

Friedman, M. J., Marmar, C. R., Baker, D. G., Sikes, C. R., & Farfel, G. M. (2007). Randomized, double-blind comparison of sertraline and placebo for posttraumatic stress disorder in a Department of Veterans Affairs setting. *Journal of Clinical Psychiatry, 68,* 711–720. doi:10.4088/JCP.v68n0508

Gunja, N. (2013). In the Zzz zone: The effects of z-drugs on human performance and driving. *Journal of Medical Toxicology, 9,* 163–171. doi:10.1007/s13181-013-0294-y

Institute of Medicine. (2007). *Treatment of posttraumatic stress disorder: An assessment of the evidence.* Washington, DC: The National Academies Press.

Ipser, J., Seedat, S., & Stein, D. J. (2006). Pharmacotherapy for post-traumatic stress disorder—a systematic review and meta-analysis: Original article. *South African Medical Journal, 96,* 1088–1096.

Kinzie, J. F., & Friedman, M. J. (2004). Psychopharmacology for refugee and asylum seeker patients. In J. P. Wilson & B. Droxdek (Eds.), *Broken spirits: The treatment of asylum seekers and refugees with PTSD* (pp. 579–600). New York, NY: Brunner-Routledge Press.

Kolb, L., Burris, B. C., & Griffiths, S. (Eds.). (1984). Propranolol and clonidine in the treatment of chronic post-traumatic stress disorders of war. In B. A. Van der Kolb (Ed.), *Post-traumatic stress disorder: Psychological and biological sequelae* (pp. 98–105). Washington, DC: American Psychiatric Press.

Kosten, T. R., Frank, J. B., Dan, E., McDougle, C. J., & Giller, E. L., Jr. (1991). Pharmacotherapy for posttraumatic stress disorder using phenelzine or imipramine. *Journal of Nervous and Mental Disease, 179,* 366–370. doi:10.1097/00005053-199106000-00011

Lindley, S. E., Carlson, E. B., & Hill, K. (2007). A randomized, double-blind, placebo-controlled trial of augmentation topiramate for chronic combat-related posttraumatic stress disorder. *Journal of Clinical Psychopharmacology, 27,* 677–681. doi:10.1097/jcp.0b013e31815a43ee

Londborg, P. D., Hegel, M. T., Goldstein, S., Goldstein, D., Himmelhoch, J. M., Maddock, R., . . . Farfel, G. M. (2001). Sertraline treatment of posttraumatic stress disorder: Results of 24 weeks of open-label continuation treatment. *Journal of Clinical Psychiatry, 62,* 325–331. doi:10.4088/JCP.v62n0503

Marshall, R. D., Beebe, K. L., Oldham, M., & Zaninelli, R. (2001). Efficacy and safety of paroxetine treatment for chronic PTSD: A fixed-dose, placebo-controlled study. *The American Journal of Psychiatry, 158,* 1982–1988. doi:10.1176/appi.ajp.158.12.1982

Marshall, R. D., Lewis-Fernández, R., Blanco C., Simpson H. B., Lin S. H., Vermes D., . . . Liebowitz M. R. (2007). A controlled trial of paroxetine for chronic PTSD, dissociation, and interpersonal problems in mostly minority adults. *Depression and Anxiety, 24,* 77–84. doi:10.1002/da.20176

Martenyi, F., Brown, E. B., & Caldwell, C. D. (2007). Failed efficacy of fluoxetine in the treatment of posttraumatic stress disorder: Results of a fixed-dose placebo-controlled study. *Journal of Clinical Psychopharmacology, 27,* 166–170. doi:10.1097/JCP.0b013e31803308ce

Martenyi, F., Brown, E. B., Zhang, H., Koke, S. C., & Prakash, A. (2002). Fluoxetine v. placebo in prevention of relapse in post-traumatic stress disorder. *The British Journal of Psychiatry, 181,* 315–320. doi:10.1192/bjp.181.4.315

Mohamed, S., & Rosenheck, R. A. (2008). Pharmacotherapy of PTSD in the U.S. Department of Veterans Affairs: Diagnostic- and symptom-guided drug selection. *Journal of Clinical Psychiatry, 69,* 959–965. doi:10.4088/JCP.v69n0611

National Institute for Clinical Excellence. (2005). *Post-traumatic stress disorder: The management of PTSD in adults and children in primary and secondary care* (Clinical Guideline 26). London, England: Author.

Petrakis, I. L., Ralevski, E., Desai, N., Trevisan, L., Gueorguieva, R., Rounsaville, B., & Krystal, J. H. (2012). Noradrenergic vs serotonergic antidepressant with or without naltrexone for veterans with PTSD and comorbid alcohol dependence. *Neuropsychopharmacology, 37,* 996–1004.

Petty, F., Fieve, R. R., Capece, J. A., & Davis, L. (2005, May). *Topiramate for civilian posttraumatic stress disorder: A pilot-controlled study.* Poster presented at the Annual Meeting of the American Psychiatric Association, Atlanta, GA.

Pollack, M. H., Hoge, E. A., Worthington, J. J., Moshier, S. J., Wechsler, R. S., Brandes, M., & Simon, N. M. (2011). Eszopiclone for the treatment of posttraumatic stress disorder and associated insomnia: A randomized, double-blind, placebo-controlled trial. *Journal of Clinical Psychiatry, 72,* 892–897. doi:10.4088/JCP.09m05607gry

Poundja, J., Sanche, S., Tremblay, J., & Brunet, A. (2012, February 14). Trauma reactivation under the influence of propranolol: An examination of clinical predictors. *European Journal of Psychotraumatology, 3.* Advance online publication. doi:10.3402/ejpt.v3i0.15470

Rapaport, M. H., Endicott, J., & Clary, C. M. (2002). Posttraumatic stress disorder and quality of life: Results across 64 weeks of sertraline treatment. *Journal of Clinical Psychiatry, 63,* 59–65. doi:10.4088/JCP.v63n0112

Raskind, M. A., Dobie, D. J., Kanter, E. D., Petrie, E. C., Thompson, C. E., Peskind, & E. R. (2000). The alpha1-adrenergic antagonist prazosin ameliorates combat trauma nightmares in veterans with posttraumatic stress disorder: A report of 4 cases. *Journal of Clinical Psychiatry, 61,* 129–133. doi:10.4088/JCP.v61n0208

Raskind, M. A., Peskind, E. R., Kanter, E. D., Petrie, E. C., Radant, A., Thompson, C. E., . . . McFall, M. M. (2003). Reduction of nightmares and other PTSD symptoms in combat veterans by prazosin: A placebo-controlled study. *The American Journal of Psychiatry, 160,* 371–373. doi:10.1176/appi.ajp.160.2.371

Raskind, M. A., Peterson, K., Williams, T., Hoff, D. J., Hart, K., Holmes, H., . . . Peskind, E. R. (2013). A trial of prazosin for combat trauma PTSD with nightmares in active-duty soldiers returned from Iraq and Afghanistan. *The American Journal of Psychiatry, 170,* 1003–1010. doi:10.1176/appi.ajp.2013.12081133

Raskind, M. A., Thompson, C., Petrie, E. C., Dobie, D. J., Rein, R. J., Hoff, D. J., . . . Peskind E. R. (2002). Prazosin reduces nightmares in combat veterans with posttraumatic stress disorder. *The Journal of Clinical Psychiatry, 63,* 565–568. doi:10.4088/JCP.v63n0705

Shalev, A. Y., Ankri, Y., Israeli-Shalev, Y., Peleg, T., Adessky, R., & Freedman, S. (2012). Prevention of posttraumatic stress disorder by early treatment: Results from the Jerusalem Trauma Outreach and Prevention study. *Archives of General Psychiatry, 69*, 166–176. doi:10.1001/archgenpsychiatry.2011.127

Shiromani, P., Keane, T. M., & LeDoux, J. E. (Eds.). (2012). *Post-traumatic stress disorder: Basic science and clinical practice.* New York, NY: Humana Press.

Stein, D. J., Ipser, J. C., & Seedat, S. (2006). Pharmacotherapy for post traumatic stress disorder (PTSD). *Cochrane Database of Systematic Reviews, 1,* CD002795.

Stein, D. J., Pedersen, R., Rothbaum, B. O, Baldwin, D. S, Ahmed, S., Musgnung, J., & Davidson, J. (2009). Onset of activity and time to response on individual CAPS-SX17 items in patients treated for post-traumatic stress disorder with venlafaxine ER: A pooled analysis. *The International Journal of Neuropsychopharmacology, 12,* 23–31.

Suris, A., North, C., Adinoff, B., Powell, C. M., & Greene, R. (2010). Effects of exogenous glucocorticoid on combat-related PTSD symptoms. *Annals of Clinical Psychiatry, 22,* 274–279.

Taylor, F., & Raskind, M. A. (2002). The alpha1-adrenergic antagonist prazosin improves sleep and nightmares in civilian trauma posttraumatic stress disorder. *Journal of Clinical Psychopharmacology, 22,* 82–85. doi:10.1097/00004714-200202000-00013

Tol, W. A., Barbui, C., & van Ommeren, M. (2013). Management of acute stress, PTSD, and bereavement: WHO recommendations. *JAMA, 310,* 477–478. doi:10.1001/jama.2013.166723

Tucker, P., Potter-Kimball, R., Wyatt, D. B., Parker, D. E., Burgin, C., Jones, D. E., & Masters, B. K. (2003). Can physiologic assessment and side effects tease out differences in PTSD trials? A double-blind comparison of citalopram, sertraline, and placebo. *Psychopharmacology Bulletin, 37,* 135–149.

Tucker, P., Trautman, R. P., Wyatt, D. B, Thompson, J., Wu, S. C., Capece, J. A., & Rosenthal, N. R. (2007). Efficacy and safety of topiramate monotherapy in civilian posttraumatic stress disorder: A randomized, double-blind, placebo-controlled study. *Journal of Clinical Psychiatry, 68,* 201–206. doi:10.4088/JCP.v68n0204

Tucker, P., Zaninelli, R., Yehuda, R., Ruggiero, L., Dillingham, K., & Pitts, C. D. (2001). Paroxetine in the treatment of chronic posttraumatic stress disorder: Results of a placebo-controlled, flexible-dosage trial. *Journal of Clinical Psychiatry, 62,* 860–868. doi:10.4088/JCP.v62n1105

U.S. Department of Veterans Affairs & Department of Defense. (2010). *VA/DoD Clinical Practice Guidelines. Management of post-traumatic stress disorder and acute stress reaction*. Retrieved from http://www.healthquality.va.gov/Post_Traumatic_Stress_Disorder_PTSD.asp

World Health Organization, Mental Health Gap Action Programme. (2013). *mhGAP intervention guide for mental, neurological and substance use disorders in non-specialized health settings*. Retrieved from http://www.ncbi.nlm.nih.gov/books/NBK138690/pdf/TOC.pdf

Yeh, M. S. L., Mari, J. J., Costa, M. C. P., Andreoli, S. B., Bressan, R. A., & Mello, M. F. (2011). A double-blind randomized controlled trial to study the efficacy of topiramate in a civilian sample of PTSD. *CNS Neuroscience & Therapeutics, 17*, 305–310. doi:10.1111/j.1755-5949.2010.00188.x

Zohar, J., Amital, D., Miodownik, C., Kotler, M., Bleich, A., Lane, R. M., & Austin, C. (2002). Double-blind placebo-controlled pilot study of sertraline in military veterans with posttraumatic stress disorder. *Journal of Clinical Psychopharmacology, 22*, 190–195. doi:10.1097/00004714-200204000-00013

5

The Use of Anxiolytics in the Management of PTSD

Nancy C. Bernardy, Tasha Souter, and Matthew J. Friedman

Anxiolytics refer to any medication that reduces symptoms of anxiety, agitation, or tension. In the past, this class of medications most commonly referred to benzodiazepines such as alprazolam (Xanax), clonazepam (Klonopin), diazepam (Valium), and lorazepam (Ativan) but now also refers to antidepressant selective serotonin reuptake inhibitors (SSRIs), such as sertraline (Zoloft) and escitalopram (Lunesta) as well as serotonin-norepinephrine reuptake inhibitors (SNRIs) such as venlafaxine (Effexor) and duloxetine (Cymbalta). These medications are included here because, with Food and Drug Administration approval of duloxetine, venlafaxine, paroxetine, and escitalopram for the treatment of generalized anxiety disorder and the increased use of SSRIs for anxiety disorders more broadly, the numbers of medications considered to have

---

Appreciation is expressed to Dr. Bruce Capehart of Durham, NC, who shared the case presentation given in this chapter.

http://dx.doi.org/10.1037/14522-006
A Practical Guide to PTSD Treatment: Pharmacological and Psychotherapeutic Approaches,
N. C. Bernardy and M. J. Friedman (Editors)
Copyright © 2015 by the American Psychological Association. All rights reserved.

anxiolytic properties have expanded. SSRIs, SNRIs, and escitalopram are reviewed in a separate chapter, however, so the primary focus here is on benzodiazepines and their role in the management of posttraumatic stress disorder (PTSD). This chapter provides an overview of the risks associated with chronic benzodiazepine use, a review of the limited research on benzodiazepines in patients with a diagnosis of PTSD, and strategies to minimize new prescriptions and taper existing ones. Alternative treatment recommendations to clinicians to address symptoms of anxiety or insomnia in those individuals who have a PTSD diagnosis are offered.

RISKS OF BENZODIAZEPINE TREATMENTS

Benzodiazepines were introduced in the 1960s as alternatives to barbiturates, which were effective as sedatives but dangerous in overdose and often abused (Lader, 2011). The stress-reducing and sedating properties of benzodiazepines made them a seemingly ideal medication to manage symptoms of anxiety and insomnia, and they became useful in addressing various clinical states such as seizures, acute alcohol withdrawal, periodic limb movements such as restless leg syndrome, and musculoskeletal spasms. By the 1970s, benzodiazepines became the most commonly prescribed class of medications in the world, but their long-term effects have gone largely unaddressed. In 2008, 85 million prescriptions were filled for the top 20 benzodiazepines, an increase of 10 million over 2004, according to IMS Health (Balestra, 2009), a health-care information company based in Connecticut.

In the 1980s, after a PTSD psychiatric diagnosis was originally established in the third edition of the *Diagnostic and Statistical Manual of Mental Disorders* (American Psychiatric Association, 1987), benzodiazepines were the primary PTSD medication, and their anxiety-reducing properties made them seem a model agent for the management of hyperarousal symptoms related to PTSD (Friedman, 1988). The term *benzodiazepines* now represents a broad class of drugs with similar pharmacological properties but differences in length of action (short-acting, intermediate, or long-acting) as well as half-life effects whether prescribed to treat anxiety or for insomnia.

One of the advantages of benzodiazepines was their early onset of action with initial anxiolytic effects noted soon after taking a first pill (Otto & Pollack, 2009). However, soon after their development and widespread use, anecdotal reports began to surface about potential withdrawal symptoms and risks of tolerance and dependence. Although typically recommended for short-term use (2–4 weeks), two thirds of U.S. prescriptions for benzodiazepines go to those who use 30 doses or more per month and are prescribed for longer periods of time (Kripke, 2000).

The known risks associated with benzodiazepines have grown in recent years. Well-recognized risks of chronic benzodiazepine use include accidents and falls, increased mortality and disinhibition-aggression, cognitive effects, and development of sleep difficulties. Concerns now include issues of impairment in learning, impairment in retention of cognitive behavioral treatment (CBT) effects, attribution of treatment gains, and medication discontinuation difficulties (Hofmann, 2012). These safety concerns have contributed to the controversy surrounding their use today.

Risks of accidents, injuries, and falls increase in those using benzodiazepines. The medication is responsible for an increase in the risk of traffic accidents by 2 to 3 times (Lader, 2011). These risks particularly increase in the elderly; benzodiazepines are responsible for a significant increase in fall rates and hip fractures in older adults (Tsunoda et al., 2010), and the rate of hip fractures increases by as much as 50% (Lader, 2011).

Long-term use of benzodiazepines has been noted to increase overall mortality rates by 50% (Kripke, 2000). The mortality hazard associated with taking prescribed sleeping pills 30 days in the previous month is similar to the hazard of smoking 1 to 2 cigarettes a day (Kripke, 2000). Recent concerns have been noted about the impact of benzodiazepines on the immune system, with increases seen in incidence of infections, mortality from sepsis, and an increased risk of pneumonia and mortality (Obiora, Hubbard, Sanders, & Myles, 2013). Finally, receipt of benzodiazepines has been related to increases in aggressive behavior among patients who were aggressive at baseline, which is a concern in some of the returning Iraq and Afghanistan veterans (Shin, Rosen, Greenbaum, & Jain, 2012).

Cognitive dysfunction has been recognized as a particularly concerning effect of benzodiazepine use. Acute and short-term administration of benzodiazepines clearly impairs higher brain functions such as learning and memory (Curran, 1986). Acquisition of new material after benzodiazepine administration (anterograde memory) is consistently impaired, with the more demands made on memory, the larger the effect (Curran, 1991). The cognitive effects improve with discontinuation of the benzodiazepine, but postwithdrawal cognitive capacity remains below nonbenzodiazepine control group norms even after 3 months off the medication. A concern has been the development of severe cognitive decline, which may be misdiagnosed as dementia. Elderly patients who had received benzodiazepines showed a 50% increased risk of dementia over never-users (Billioti de Gage et al., 2012). The cognitive effects from chronic benzodiazepine use are of particular concern in the veteran PTSD population. PTSD itself is a risk factor for dementia, with rates in older veterans with PTSD as high as 2 times those without PTSD (Yaffe et al., 2010). There are also high rates of co-occurring traumatic brain injury or postconcussive syndrome in the veteran PTSD population, and benzodiazepines are contraindicated in this group.

The recognized effects of chronic benzodiazepine use on sleep are interesting because they are often prescribed to treat insomnia. Benzodiazepines decrease sleep-onset latency, decrease Stage 1 sleep, increase Stage 2 and 3 sleep, increase rapid eye movement (REM) latency, and increase total REM sleep (Holbrook, Crowther, Lotter, Cheng, & King, 2000). Although initially effective with insomnia, tolerance to the hypnotic effect occurs within days to weeks of regular use, and the benefits of the benzodiazepine dissolve by 1 to 5 weeks of chronic use (Lader, 2011). Patients often report continued benefit, possibly due to prevention of rebound insomnia. Patients also often believe that a sleeping pill will improve their daytime functioning, despite evidence that these medications consistently impair performance, cognition, and memory. Benzodiazepines are contraindicated when clinical concerns such as chronic obstructive pulmonary disease or obstructive sleep apnea are present.

In the treatment of other mental health disorders in which benzodiazepines have previously been indicated (e.g., panic disorder, generalized anxiety disorder), there is increasing recognition that CBT alone is superior to benzodiazepines alone. Concurrent benzodiazepines lead to increased dropout rates, attenuated short-term gains, and reduced long-term benefit of CBT (Westra & Stewart, 1998). More significant effects are seen with high-potency benzodiazepines, likely because of their effect on state-dependent learning (Bouton, Kenney, & Rosengard, 1990). Some of these factors may also be related to the previously mentioned memory effects—the anterograde amnestic effects. In PTSD, benzodiazepines may interfere with the mental processes necessary to fully benefit from psychotherapy (van Minnen, Arntz, & Keijsers, 2002). This is thought to be especially prominent with daytime dosing and with long-acting benzodiazepines.

Patterns of prescribed benzodiazepine use are linked to demographic, lifestyle, and clinical variables. Internationally the majority of benzodiazepine prescriptions are written for those who are over 30, White, well educated, and female. Sleep disturbances and smoking have also been associated with higher receipt of benzodiazepines (Nordfjaern et al., 2014). Female veterans with PTSD have been found to receive prescribed benzodiazepines at increasing rates compared with male veterans with PTSD, among whom recent rates have decreased (Bernardy et al., 2013). It is unknown whether this is due to greater diagnostic frequency or increased comorbid conditions or whether other reasons, such as gender differences in acceptance and receipt of mental health treatment, contribute to this prescribing difference.

An important consideration for women of childbearing age is that although benzodiazepines are frequently used in postpartum women to control anxiety, panic disorder, and seizures, the risk of breastfeeding while taking these drugs remains a controversial and underresearched topic. As a rule, drugs in the benzodiazepine family are not ideal for breastfeeding (Malone, Papagni, Ramini, & Keltner, 2004). Any time an infant is exposed to a benzodiazepine, monitoring for central nervous system depression and apnea is advised. Another concern is that women of childbearing age who take benzodiazepines are more likely to report no use of contraception and thus are at risk of unintended pregnancy but are unaware of the teratogenic risks associated with benzodiazepine use (Schwarz et al., 2013).

Because benzodiazepines are frequently used in conjunction with other drugs, polysedative use is a prominent problem. Among 20,041 patients with PTSD, preexisting diagnosis of drug abuse increased the risk of being prescribed very high daily doses of benzodiazepines for extended periods of time (Hermos, Young, Lawler, Rosenbloom, & Fiore, 2007). Being prescribed a high-dose benzodiazepine was associated with a simultaneous oxycodone prescription. Operation Iraqi Freedom/Operation Enduring Freedom veterans with PTSD are significantly more likely to receive opiates for pain, higher doses of opiates, two or more opiates, and sedative hypnotics concurrent with opiates, as well as to obtain early refills (Seal et al., 2012). Other work has found that 47% of veterans with PTSD taking benzodiazepines were concurrently prescribed long-term opioids (Hawkins, Malte, Imel, Saxon, & Kivlahan, 2012). More recent work has noted an increasing prevalence of concurrent sedatives in veterans with PTSD, with the most common combination of an opioid plus a benzodiazepine taken concurrently increasing by 15.9% (Bernardy, Lund, Alexander, & Friedman, 2013). These important trends in polysedative use among veterans with PTSD illustrate the complexity of treating a group of symptoms that best respond to sedative medications such as chronic pain and insomnia.

EVIDENCE BEHIND THE RECOMMENDATIONS REGARDING BENZODIAZEPINES IN PTSD

Research in both animals and humans suggests that benzodiazepines may interfere with the extinction of fear conditioning or potentiate the acquisition of fear responses. This action could actually worsen recovery from trauma and interfere with one of the first-line recommended PTSD psychotherapies, which include prolonged exposure therapy or cognitive processing therapy (U.S. Department of Veterans Affairs & Department of Defense [VA/DoD], 2010).

Two small clinical trials (Braun, Greenberg, Dasberg, & Lerer, 1990; Cates, Bishop, Davis, Lowe, & Woolley, 2004) tested the relative efficacy of benzodiazepines in PTSD. The first used alprazolam and showed no benefit in relieving PTSD symptoms compared with placebo (Braun et al., 1990). A small reduction in anxiety symptoms was offset by withdrawal effects after only a period of 5 weeks on the benzodiazepine. The other trial compared clonazepam with placebo for PTSD-related sleep problems and found no difference between the benzodiazepines and placebo (Cates et al., 2004). Although it was a small study, it was important because the use of benzodiazepines for sleep management in PTSD is often the clinical reason for their use. Approximately 64% of returning veterans endorse insomnia as a major complaint (Amin, Parisi, Parisi, Gold, & Gold, 2010), and efforts to address appropriate sleep care are prominent now in the treatment of veterans (Karlin, Trockel, Taylor, Gimeno, & Manber, 2013). Although widely prescribed for sleep dysfunction in PTSD (Jain, Greenbaum, & Rosen, 2012a), evidence for positive effects on PTSD-related sleep disturbances in PTSD is generally disappointing, with ill effects noted through changes in sleep architecture and poor sleep overall (Lader, 2011). See Chapter 8, this volume, for further discussion of treatment of PTSD-related sleep disruption.

Benzodiazepines have also been studied to determine if their use could acutely prevent the development of PTSD. In an open-label study (Gelpin, Bonne, Peri, Brandes, & Shalev, 1996), 13 patients who had recently experienced trauma (within the previous 18 days) and were experiencing excessive distress (panic, agitation, or persistent insomnia) were treated for up to 6 months with alprazolam or clonazepam. These patients were compared with a control group of recently traumatized individuals matched for demographics and symptoms (using the Impact of Events Scale). PTSD occurred at a significantly higher rate in the benzodiazepine-treated group (nine of 13, 69%) than in the control group (two of 13, 15%) at follow-up. The study suggested that benzodiazepines may worsen outcomes in the acute period after trauma, and the authors referenced animal data consistent with the hypothesis that benzodiazepines may potentiate the acquisition of fear responses.

A double-blind randomized controlled study (Mellman, Bustamante, David, & Fins, 2002) was then conducted during the acute period after trauma (mean 2 weeks after trauma). Short-term (7 day) evening use of temazepam in patients with significant acute stress disorder or PTSD symptoms was compared with placebo (11 patients in each group). The study showed no benefits in preventing PTSD, and the trend was similar to the Gelpin (1996) study, with six of 11 (55%) patients who received temazepam developing PTSD, compared with three of 11 (27%) who received placebo. Finally, Davydow, Gifford, Desai, Needham, and Bienvenu (2008), in a literature review of the risk factors for developing PTSD after serious trauma (requiring intensive care unit [ICU] treatment), found that greater benzodiazepine administration in the ICU was one of the consistent predictors of PTSD.

CURRENT GUIDELINE RECOMMENDATIONS REGARDING BENZODIAZEPINE USE

Various clinical practice guidelines do not support the use of benzodiazepines for the pharmacologic management of PTSD (Jain, Greenbaum, & Rosen, 2012b). The VA/DoD (2010) Clinical Practice Guideline, the American Psychiatric Association (Ursano et al., 2004), and the International Society for Traumatic Stress Studies (Foa, Keane, Friedman, & Cohen, 2009) all caution clinicians about prescribing benzodiazepines, citing lack of efficacy data for core PTSD symptoms and safety concerns, particularly in patients with a history of substance use disorders. The research supporting this recommendation is, however, limited. Currently no data support the efficacy of benzodiazepines for the management of the core PTSD symptoms that include avoidance, hyperarousal, numbing, or dissociation. Previously it was thought that the use of benzodiazepines in patients with PTSD was intended to treat a co-occurring diagnosis in which their use would be indicated, such as with panic disorder or other anxiety disorders. More recent research points to their probable nonindicated use to manage symptoms of chronic insomnia (Bernardy, Lund, Alexander, & Friedman, 2012; Jain et al., 2012a). With the development of newer and safer medications such as the SSRIs and the SNRIs, as well as changes in anxiety disorder treatment recommendations that promote the use of SSRIs in conjunction with CBT and the development of newer medications, such as prazosin and escitalopram, and CBT for insomnia (CBT–I), the debate about the continued use of benzodiazepines has reopened (Bernardy, 2013).

These studies contributed to the decision of the PTSD Clinical Practice Guideline Workgroup to strongly recommend against the use of benzodiazepines to prevent the development of acute stress disorder or PTSD (VA/DoD, 2010). The guideline notes that a short-term course of benzodiazepines can be effective against anxiety and insomnia but that these medications should be used with caution in patients with acute stress disorder and PTSD because of the high frequency of co-occurring substance abuse and dependence in patients with PTSD. The balance between benefit and potential risks, including the risks of dependency and of withdrawal after discontinuation, should be evaluated when considering benzodiazepines in patients with acute stress reaction.

PRESCRIBING RECOMMENDATIONS FOR BENZODIAZEPINES

Despite the lack of efficacy data and increasing concerns about safety, benzodiazepines are still widely used in the management of PTSD. Research in civilian populations has noted rates of approximately 40% of individuals with PTSD were prescribed a benzodiazepine. In recent work examining their use in veteran populations, a decreased rate of 30% from 36% a decade earlier has been observed (Jain et al., 2012b; Lund, Bernardy, Bernardy, Alexander & Friedman, 2012), but that percentage is set against a backdrop of a rapidly increasing number of veterans diagnosed with PTSD, so the actual number of veterans prescribed benzodiazepines has increased sharply. This suggests that the continued widespread use of benzodiazepines in the treatment of PTSD is not based on research evidence and that a targeted intervention may be necessary to achieve further reduction in the use of these agents.

Suggested strategies for minimizing new benzodiazepine prescriptions for anxiety include a discussion between the provider and the patient that benzodiazepines are for symptom control only and do not improve PTSD symptoms over time (Cloos & Ferreira, 2009). Education regarding the relationship between PTSD and substance use and PTSD-related avoidance should help, and education regarding the associated risks of long-term use is critical. Providers should assess for cognitive impairments and ask about a history of traumatic brain injury. A comprehensive assessment of substance use, including a random urine drug screen, should take place. For any new prescriptions, a clinician should develop a clearly outlined treatment plan to target PTSD with first-line treatment options including SSRI or SNRIs, CBT, or adjunctive treatment using prazosin for trauma-related nightmares. If prescribed, adhere to short-term (2–4 weeks) indication. Generally, use 50% doses in elderly patients and avoid as much as possible doing even that.

Strategies for minimizing new prescriptions for sleep should include an assessment for primary sleep disorders and a referral for a sleep study. Depression and any existing substance use disorder should be treated. Intake of nicotine and stimulants including caffeine should be determined as should a review of sleep hygiene. Excellent options for non-benzodiazepine sleep agents include trazodone, mirtazapine, and tricyclic antidepressants. Benadryl and hydroxyzine are other options but should be avoided in patients with cognitive impairment and those with a history of mild traumatic brain injury. Atypical antipsychotics such as low-dose quetiapine should be avoided for sleep alone. Consider prazosin, which is effective for reducing trauma-related nightmares and improving sleep quality (Raskind et al., 2013). CBT–I has components that include stimulus control, sleep restriction, cognitive therapy, relaxation techniques, and sleep hygiene education. CBT–I has been shown to be superior to pharmacotherapy at 8 weeks and more effective long-term than pharmacotherapy (Karlin et al., 2013).

Strategies for tapering existing prescriptions include establishing a stable relationship between patient and provider. Evaluate and treat any co-occurring medical and psychiatric conditions. Obtain complete drug and alcohol history and random drug screen. Review recent medical notes (emergency room visits, primary care providers, other providers, prescriptions and medication lists, refill requests) and coordinate care with other providers. If it is available in your area, consider querying state prescription drug monitoring databases.

Simple strategies for tapering existing prescriptions include the following: a single letter from a primary care provider urging gradual reduction and perhaps in time, cessation of benzodiazepine use led to two thirds reduction in dosage at 6 months (Lader, 2011). Brief advice during a consultation and a self-help booklet led to 18% of patients reducing their dosages versus 5% in the control group. Initiating provider audits and limits such as only a 30-day supply and in-person refills have been shown to reduce benzodiazepine prescriptions by as much as 50%.

For complex cases, it is critical that the provider be flexible with a taper schedule. Yet a prolonged taper of over 6 months may actually worsen the long-term outcomes. It is suggested that providers consider stabilizing the patient on 50% dose for several months before proceeding with a taper. One helpful consideration is to switch to long-acting benzodiazepines. This can be particularly helpful with alprazolam tapers, with long-term users or those on supratherapeutic doses or short half-life benzodiazepines. Residential treatment can be of support, and a team of providers that offer support to the patient, including a case manager, clinical pharmacist, therapist, and primary care provider, can be effective.

CURRENTLY FAVORED TREATMENTS

Concurrent CBT has also been shown to be effective with tapering of existing prescriptions. In patients with panic disorder, those who received group CBT during a slow taper had 76% success, versus 25% with slow taper alone. CBT–I concurrent with taper has shown improved outcomes (Otto et al., 1993).

There are specific patient groups that providers might want to prioritize for efforts to taper existing benzodiazepine prescriptions. Patients who are on multiple benzodiazepines or are on combinations of benzodiazepines with opioids or prescribed amphetamines should be a priority group because of safety concerns of the combination of medications. Any patients with an active (or a history of) substance abuse or dependence should be prioritized, as should anyone with a cognitive disorder or a history of mild traumatic brain injury. Elderly patients are another group at increased risk of injury or adverse cognitive effects from these medications. Caution should be taken with women of childbearing age. Finally, younger military veterans should be prioritized because they can have better long-term treatment outcomes using SSRIs and evidence-based cognitive behavioral psychotherapies.

CASE STUDY

The following case presentation illustrates the complexity of tapering a patient from chronic benzodiazepines. Jim is a Vietnam veteran who has taken benzodiazepines since the late 1980s and is now in his mid-60s. He was an infantryman with a lot of combat experience, witnessed significant stressors, and suffered rocket fire wounds. He came to a Veterans Affairs psychiatrist with a great deal of experience in PTSD clinics in 2009. He was angry, irritable, and did not want treatment but needed to discuss his PTSD to continue to get benefits. At the initial meeting, he had completed many trials of tricyclic antidepressants, different SSRIs, and bupropion but felt that alprazolam 0.5 mg taken four times daily was the only thing that kept his anger in check. It took a long time for the psychiatrist to build a therapeutic relationship with Jim. He continued to take his benzodiazepine while the provider talked to him about considering another antidepressant. After several discussions of nefazodone as a possible treatment, he consented to a trial. Within 6 months, a marked improvement in his PTSD symptoms was observed. He began to cut back on the alprazolam on his own, taking it as needed for acute anxiety. The combination of nefazodone with insight into his anger and irritability allowed him to practice what he wanted to say before encounters with people, leading to greatly reduced anxiety. He developed concerns, however, about continued use of nefazodone and now manages his anxiety with sertraline and has stopped taking the alprazolam. He was not eager to do so, but given his increasing concerns about his need for long-term care as he gets older, he was finally able to stop taking the medication.

CONCLUSION

In summary, investigators have made remarkable progress in developing efficacious first-line recommended interventions for PTSD. Clinicians should determine whether patients who have "failed" previous pharmacological treatments received an adequate trial. It may be the case that another SSRI trial to get the patient to a therapeutic level should be tried or one of the newer SNRIs be prescribed. Because of the significant risks associated with benzodiazepines and the lack of evidence for their effectiveness in the treatment of PTSD, it is worthwhile to implement strategies to carefully assess and consider alternative treatment options as well as to minimize new benzodiazepine prescriptions whenever possible. Despite the involved challenges, strategies to taper existing benzodiazepine prescriptions can be effective.

REFERENCES

American Psychiatric Association. (1987). *Diagnostic and statistical manual of mental disorders* (3rd ed.; text rev.). Washington, DC: Author.

Amin, M. M., Parisi, J. A., Gold, M. S., & Gold, A. R. (2010). War-related illness symptoms among Operation Iraqi Freedom/Operation Enduring Freedom returnees. *Military Medicine, 175*, 155–157. doi:10.7205/MILMED-D-09-00153

Balestra, K. (2009, June 30). Critics cite serious side effects of benzodiazepine antidepressants. *The Washington Post*. Retrieved from http://www.washingtonpost.com/wp-dyn/content/article/2009/06/29/AR2009062903105.html

Bernardy, N. C. (2013). The role of benzodiazepines in the treatment of posttraumatic stress disorder (PTSD). *PTSD Research Quarterly, 23*, 1–9.

Bernardy, N. C., Lund, B. C., Alexander, B., & Friedman, M. J. (2012). Prescribing trends in veterans with posttraumatic stress disorder. *Journal of Clinical Psychiatry, 73*, 297–303.

Bernardy, N. C., Lund, B. C., Alexander, B., & Friedman, M. J. (2013, December 16). Increased polysedative use in veterans with posttraumatic stress disorder. *Pain Medicine.* Advance publication online. doi:10.1111/pme.12321

Bernardy, N. C., Lund, B. C., Alexander, B., Jenkyn, A. B., Schnurr, P. P., & Friedman, M. J. (2013). Gender differences in prescribing among veterans diagnosed with posttraumatic stress disorder. *Journal of General Internal Medicine, 28*(Suppl. 2), S542–S548. doi:10.1007/s11606-012-2260-9

Billioti de Gage, S., Bégaud, B., Bazin, F., Verdoux, H., Dartigues, J.-F., Pérès, K., . . . Pariente, A. (2012). Benzodiazepine use and risk of dementia: Prospective population based study. *BMJ: British Medical Journal, 345,* e6231. doi:10.1136/bmj.e6231

Bouton, M. E., Kenney, F. A., & Rosengard, C. (1990). State-dependent fear extinction with two benzodiazepine tranquilizers. *Behavioral Neuroscience, 104,* 44–55. doi:10.1037/0735-7044.104.1.44

Braun, P., Greenberg, D., Dasberg, H., & Lerer, B. (1990). Core symptoms of posttraumatic stress disorder unimproved by alprazolam treatment. *Journal of Clinical Psychiatry, 51,* 236–238.

Cates, M. E., Bishop, M. H., Davis, L. L., Lowe, J. S., & Woolley, T. W. (2004). Clonazepam for treatment of sleep disturbances associated with combat-related posttraumatic stress disorder. *The Annals of Pharmacotherapy, 38,* 1395–1399. doi:10.1345/aph.1E043

Cloos, J. M., & Ferreira, V. (2009). Current use of benzodiazepines in anxiety disorders. *Current Opinion in Psychiatry, 22,* 90–95. doi:10.1097/YCO.0b013e32831a473d

Curran, H. V. (1986). Tranquillising memories: A review of the effects of benzodiazepines on human memory. *Biological Psychology, 23,* 179–213. doi:10.1016/0301-0511(86)90081-5

Curran, H. V. (1991). Benzodiazepines, memory and mood: A review. *Psychopharmacology, 105,* 1–8. doi:10.1007/BF02316856

Davydow, D. S., Gifford, J. M., Desai, S. V., Needham, D. M., & Bienvenu, O. J. (2008). Posttraumatic stress disorder in general intensive care unit survivors: A systematic review. *General Hospital Psychiatry, 30,* 421–434. doi:10.1016/j.genhosppsych.2008.05.006

Foa, E. B., Keane, T. M., Friedman, M. J., & Cohen, J. A. (Eds.). (2009). *Effective treatments for PTSD: Practice guidelines from the International Society for Traumatic Stress Studies* (2nd ed.). New York, NY: Guilford Press.

Friedman, M. J. (1988). Toward rational pharmacotherapy for posttraumatic stress disorder: An interim report. *The American Journal of Psychiatry, 145,* 281–285.

Gelpin, E., Bonne, O. B., Peri, T., Brandes, D., & Shalev, A. Y. (1996). Treatment of recent trauma survivors with benzodiazepines: A prospective study. *Journal of Clinical Psychiatry, 57*, 390–394.

Hawkins, E. J., Malte, C. A., Imel, Z. E., Saxon, A. J., & Kivlahan, D. R. (2012). Prevalence and trends of benzodiazepine use among Veterans Affairs patients with posttraumatic stress disorder, 2003–2010. *Drug and Alcohol Dependence, 124*, 154–161. doi:10.1016/j.drugalcdep.2012.01.003

Hermos, J. A., Young, M. M., Lawler, E. V., Rosenbloom, D., & Fiore, L. D. (2007). Long-term, high-dose benzodiazepine prescriptions in veteran patients with PTSD: Influence of preexisting alcoholism and drug-abuse diagnoses. *Journal of Traumatic Stress, 20*, 909–914. doi:10.1002/jts.20254

Hofmann, S. G. (Ed.). (2012). *Psychobiological approaches for anxiety disorders: Treatment combination strategies* (Wiley Series in Clinical Psychology). Manchester, England: Wiley-Blackwell.

Holbrook, A. M., Crowther, R., Lotter, A, Cheng, C., & King, D. (2000). Meta-analysis of benzodiazepine use in the treatment of insomnia. *Canadian Medical Association Journal, 162*, 225–233.

Jain, S., Greenbaum, M. A., & Rosen, C. S. (2012a). Concordance between psychotropic prescribing for veterans with PTSD and clinical practice guidelines. *Psychiatric Services, 63*, 154–160. doi:10.1176/appi.ps.201100199

Jain, S., Greenbaum, M. A., & Rosen, C. S. (2012b, March 8). Do veterans with posttraumatic stress disorder receive first-line pharmacotherapy? Results from the longitudinal veterans health survey. *The Primary Care Companion to CNS Disorders, 14*(2). Advance online publication. doi:10.4088/PCC.

Karlin, B. E., Trockel, M., Taylor, M., Gimeno, J., & Manber, R. (2013). National dissemination of cognitive behavioral therapy for insomnia in veterans: Therapist- and patient-level outcomes. *Journal of Consulting and Clinical Psychology, 81*, 912–917. doi:10.1037/a0032554

Kripke, D. F. (2000). Chronic hypnotic use: Deadly risks, doubtful benefit. *Sleep Medicine Reviews, 4*, 5–20. doi:10.1053/smrv.1999.0076

Lader, M. (2011). Benzodiazepines revisited—will we ever learn? *Addiction, 106*, 2086–2109. doi:10.1111/j.1360-0443.2011.03563.x

Lund, B. C., Bernardy, N. C., Alexander B., & Friedman, M. J. (2012). Declining benzodiazepine use in veterans with posttraumatic stress disorder. *Journal of Clinical Psychiatry, 73*, 292–296.

Malone, K., Papagni, K., Ramini, S., & Keltner, N. L. (2004). Antidepressants, antipsychotics, benzodiazepines, and the breastfeeding dyad. *Perspectives in Psychiatric Care, 40*, 73–85. doi:10.1111/j.1744-6163.2004.00073.x

Mellman, T. A., Bustamante, V., David, D., & Fins, A. I. (2002). Hypnotic medication in the aftermath of trauma [letter]. *Journal of Clinical Psychiatry, 63,* 1183–1184. doi:10.4088/JCP.v63n1214h

Nordfjaern, T., Bjerkeset, O., Bratberg, G., Moylan, S, Berk, M., & Gråwe, R. (2014). Socio-demographic, lifestyle and psychological predictors of benzodiazepine and z-hypnotic use patterns. *Nordic Journal of Psychiatry, 68,* 107–116.

Obiora, E., Hubbard, R., Sanders, R. D., & Myles, P. R. (2013). The impact of benzodiazepines on occurrence of pneumonia and mortality from pneumonia: A nested case–control and survival analysis in a population-based cohort. *Thorax, 68,* 163–170. doi:10.1136/thoraxjnl-2012-202374

Otto, M. W., & Pollack, M. H. (2009). *Stopping anxiety medication.* New York, NY: Oxford University Press.

Otto, M. W., Pollack, M. H., Sachs, G. S., Reiter, S. R., Meltzer-Brody, S., & Rosenbaum, J. F. (1993). Discontinuation of benzodiazepine treatment: Efficacy of cognitive-behavioral therapy for patients with panic disorder. *The American Journal of Psychiatry, 150,* 1485–1490.

Raskind, M. A., Peterson, K., Williams, T., Hoff, D. J., Hart, K., Holmes, H., . . . Peskind, E. R. (2013). A trial of prazosin for combat trauma PTSD with nightmares in active-duty soldiers returned from Iraq and Afghanistan. *The American Journal of Psychiatry, 170,* 1003–1010. doi:10.1176/appi.ajp.2013.12081133

Schwarz, E. B., Mattocks, K., Brandt, C., Borrero, S., Zephyrin, L. C., Bathulapalli, H., & Haskell, S. (2013). Counseling of female veterans about risks of medication-induced birth defects. *Journal of General Internal Medicine, 28*(Suppl. 2), S598–S603. doi:10.1007/s11606-012-2240-0

Seal, K. H., Shi, Y., Cohen, G., Cohen, B. E., Maguen, S., Krebs, E. E., & Neylan, T. C. (2012). Association of mental health disorders with prescription opioids and high-risk opioid use in US Veterans of Iraq and Afghanistan. *JAMA, 307,* 940–947. doi:10.1001/jama.2012.234

Shin, H. J., Rosen, C. S., Greenbaum, M. A., & Jain, S. (2012). Longitudinal correlates of aggressive behavior in help-seeking U.S. veterans with PTSD. *Journal of Traumatic Stress, 25,* 649–656. doi:10.1002/jts.21761

Tsunoda, K., Uchida, H., Suzuki, T., Watanabe, K., Yamashima, T., & Kashima, H. (2010). Effects of discontinuing benzodiazepine-derivative hypnotics on postural sway and cognitive functions in the elderly. *International Journal of Geriatric Psychiatry, 25,* 1259–1265. doi:10.1002/gps.2465

Ursano, R. J., Bell, C. C., Eth, S., Friedman, M., Norwood, A., Pfefferbaum, B., . . . Steering Committee on Practice Guidelines. (2004). Practice guideline for the treatment of acute stress and posttraumatic stress disorder. *The American Journal of Psychiatry, 161*(Suppl. 11), 3–31.

U.S. Department of Veterans Affairs & U.S. Department of Defense. (2010, October). *VA/DoD Clinical Practice Guidelines. Management of post-traumatic stress disorder and acute stress reaction*. Retrieved from http://www.healthquality.va.gov/Post_Traumatic_Stress_Disorder_PTSD.asp

van Minnen, A., Arntz, A., & Keijsers, G. P. (2002). Prolonged exposure in patients with chronic PTSD: Predictors of treatment outcome and dropout. *Behaviour Research and Therapy, 40*, 439–457. doi:10.1016/S0005-7967(01)00024-9

Westra, H. A., & Stewart, S. H. (1998). Cognitive behavioural therapy and pharmacotherapy: Complementary or contradictory approaches to the treatment of anxiety? *Clinical Psychology Review, 18*, 307–340. doi:10.1016/S0272-7358(97)00084-6

Yaffe, K., Vittinghoff, E., Lindquist, K., Barnes, D., Covinsky, K. E., Neylan, T., . . . Marmar, C. (2010). Posttraumatic stress disorder and risk of dementia among U.S. veterans. *Archives of General Psychiatry, 67*, 608–613. doi:10.1001/archgenpsychiatry.2010.61

6

Atypical Antipsychotics and Anticonvulsants in the Treatment of PTSD: Treatment Options That Include Cognitive Behavioral Therapies

Matthew D. Jeffreys

With limited medication options available for treating posttraumatic stress disorder (PTSD), there has been a growing interest in second-line agents that might address the core PTSD symptoms of reexperiencing, hyperarousal, and avoidance. This is especially true for patients who are refractory to the selective serotonin reuptake inhibitors (SSRIs) and the selective serotonin/norepinephrine reuptake inhibitor (SNRI) venlafaxine, which are recommended first-line agents in PTSD clinical practice guidelines (Foa, Keane, Friedman, & Cohen, 2009; U.S. Department of Veterans Affairs & Department of Defense, 2010). The atypical antipsychotics and the anticonvulsants are frequently used off-label treatments for PTSD despite limited data to support their use.

Clinicians are often confronted with complex presentations of PTSD, including comorbid mood and substance use disorders that may include psychotic features. It is important to differentiate the core PTSD

http://dx.doi.org/10.1037/14522-007
A Practical Guide to PTSD Treatment: Pharmacological and Psychotherapeutic Approaches,
N. C. Bernardy and M. J. Friedman (Editors)
Copyright © 2015 by the American Psychological Association. All rights reserved.

symptoms being targeted from the comorbid conditions for which the atypical antipsychotics and anticonvulsants have a more established role. This chapter explores the rationale for their use, along with concerns about their side effects and efficacy. Only randomized, placebo-controlled trials are considered.

ATYPICAL ANTIPSYCHOTICS

The benefits of drugs targeting the serotonergic system are well known in PTSD. Because of their relatively greater activity at the serotonin receptor compared with first-generation agents, atypical antipsychotics have been of interest in PTSD treatment. In addition, sleep is a common problem in PTSD, and these agents may promote sleep through their blockade of the histamine receptor. They also block the alpha-1 receptor, as does prazosin, so their effect on nightmares is of interest (Tripathi & Macaluso, 2013). Finally, these agents have been used to decrease agitation in a number of disorders, including psychosis, bipolar disorder, and delirium, so there has been interest in their effect on decreasing hyperarousal in PTSD.

Risperidone and olanzapine are the only atypical or second-generation antipsychotics to date with randomized controlled trials regarding their efficacy in PTSD. This section provides a brief review of the current literature regarding their use in treating PTSD.

The only study of risperidone monotherapy demonstrated significantly decreased Treatment Outcome for PTSD—8 and total Clinician Administered PTSD Scale (CAPS) scores compared with placebo (Padala et al., 2006). Risperidone has been evaluated as adjunctive treatment for PTSD in five randomized controlled trials. Three of these trials showed positive benefit, and two showed no benefit in treating PTSD symptoms. Studies that were positive showed decreased levels of irritable aggression, hyperarousal, and reexperiencing symptoms as evidenced by lowering the total score on the CAPS and the PTSD Checklist (Bartzokis, Lu, Turner, Mintz, & Saunders, 2005; Hamner et al., 2003;

Monnelly, Ciraulo, Knapp, & Keane, 2003; Reich, Winternitz, Hennen, Watts, & Stanculescu, 2004).

The negative studies for risperidone augmentation of existing medications did not demonstrate overall reductions in PTSD measures such as the CAPS, but one study demonstrated improvement in sleep disturbance (Rothbaum et al., 2008). This finding is particularly important because clinicians might be targeting refractory sleep problems, although patients might actually benefit more from agents other than atypical antipsychotics, such as prazosin (Byers, Allison, Wendel, & Lee, 2010).

The other negative study of risperidone should receive special emphasis because it was the only large, multicenter trial comparing risperidone augmentation to placebo. Two hundred and forty-seven veterans contributed to the outcome analysis. There was no significant difference in the total CAPS score for the placebo versus risperidone group. There were statistically significant reductions on the reexperiencing and hyperarousal subscales of the CAPS consistent with other studies, but these were not clinically significant. The authors cautioned that further large-scale studies in women and nonveterans are needed (Krystal et al., 2011).

Three studies have examined the use of olanzapine in treating PTSD. The first compared olanzapine with placebo as monotherapy and demonstrated no significant difference between them, but there was a high placebo response rate (Butterfield et al., 2001). The second study compared olanzapine with placebo for augmentation of SSRI-resistant PTSD symptoms. There was a decrease in total CAPS and decrease in sleep problems. The measurement of clinical global response was not significantly different in the treatment group (Stein, Kline, & Matloff, 2002). The third study compared olanzapine with placebo as monotherapy for PTSD symptoms. There was a significant decrease in the total CAPS and on the avoidance and numbing subscales. Weight gain in the olanzapine group was substantial compared with the placebo group, however. The authors recommended larger controlled trials for olanzapine in the treatment of PTSD (Carey, Suliman, Ganesan, Seedat, & Stein, 2012).

ANTICONVULSANTS IN THE TREATMENT OF PTSD

Anticonvulsants enhance the inhibitory neurotransmitter gamma-aminobutyric acid (GABA) in the central nervous system through several mechanisms including stimulating the GABA receptor directly and inhibiting the effects of the excitatory neurotransmitter glutamate at its receptors. The concept of kindling, in which repeated stimulation to the anxiety centers of the brain (e.g., amygdala) increases sensitivity to trigger stimuli, has increased interest in using anticonvulsants to treat PTSD. Randomized, placebo-controlled trials have been completed for topiramate, lamotrigine, divalproex, and tiagabine.

Two double-blind, placebo-controlled trials have evaluated topiramate monotherapy in civilians. In the first trial, the total CAPS score decreased more in the topiramate group than in the control group but did not reach statistical significance. The hyperarousal subscale of the CAPS did decrease significantly in the treatment group, however (Tucker et al., 2007). The second study demonstrated significant reductions in reexperiencing symptoms, avoidance symptoms, and total CAPS score (Yeh et al., 2011).

Two additional double-blind, placebo-controlled studies evaluated topiramate in veterans. One study of adjunctive topiramate therapy demonstrated significant reductions in total CAPS scores and reexperiencing and hyperarousal scores for the topiramate group (Akuchekian & Amanat, 2004). A second study of topiramate monotherapy demonstrated no significant difference in total CAPS scores between the placebo and topiramate groups. However, there was a significantly greater improvement in a measure of the reexperiencing subscale of the CAPS. The authors expressed concerned about the effect of high dropout rates on the study findings (Lindley, Carlson, & Hill, 2007).

Lamotrigine was studied in 15 individuals with combat and noncombat traumas and demonstrated statistically greater improvement in the Duke Global Rating for PTSD—Improvement for both the total score and all three symptom clusters. The authors recommended larger trials for lamotrigine (Hertzberg et al., 1999).

The studies on divalproex and tiagabine have been negative for PTSD. Divalproex demonstrated no significant differences on total CAPS score or subscales. The authors demonstrated therapeutic blood levels in the trial (Davis et al., 2008). Tiagabine was studied in 232 patients with a wide variety of trauma types. This multicenter trial demonstrated no statistically significant improvement in total CAPS scores and other measures of well-being, such as the Sheehan Disability Scale for the tiagabine group (Davidson, Brady, Mellman, Stein, & Pollack, 2007).

ADDRESSING SYMPTOMS THROUGH COGNITIVE BEHAVIORAL THERAPY

Evidence-based, trauma-focused psychotherapy has been identified as a treatment of choice to address PTSD symptoms and both cognitive processing therapy (CPT) and prolonged exposure (PE) therapy have shown benefit in treating PTSD symptoms in both civilians and veterans in randomized, controlled trials (Monson et al., 2006; Resick, Nishith, Weaver, Astin, & Feuer, 2002; Schnurr et al., 2007). Skills training in affect and interpersonal regulation may enhance outcomes for patients with histories of early onset of abuse and difficulty modulating emotions (Cloitre et al., 2010). Other therapies, such as cognitive behavioral therapy (CBT) for sleep, have shown benefit for specific symptoms such as sleep disturbance in PTSD, which may be refractory at times to CPT or PE (Schoenfeld, Deviva, & Manber, 2012).

There are many advantages to psychotherapy as the primary treatment modality, including its safety, lack of medication side effects, improved sense of self-regulation, and lasting effects. Some patients may be refractory to these treatments or prefer pharmacotherapy, so a full understanding of the risk–benefit ratio and treatment options for pharmacotherapy is essential. Also, it can be challenging to find therapists who are adequately trained in CPT or PE, which may limit the available treatment options. A full description of these therapies is beyond the scope of this chapter, and the reader is referred to the cited articles for a more complete discussion and description of their use.

CASE EXAMPLE

The following fictitious case example illustrates some of the treatment dilemmas often encountered in off-label prescribing with PTSD.

The patient is a 26-year-old married White female with PTSD related to childhood abuse and comorbid bipolar disorder, type I. She is medically healthy and is using birth control. Current medications are divalproex and lamotrigine. Her past mental health history is remarkable for a hospitalization in her early 20s for a manic episode. She has never engaged in psychotherapy for PTSD. There is a positive family history of bipolar disorder in the patient's mother. She has a stable living situation currently with her husband and does not work. She consults a private psychiatrist regarding her ongoing PTSD symptoms. The psychiatrist begins sertraline as a Food and Drug Administration (FDA)-approved medication for PTSD and discusses with the patient the risk of the SSRI precipitating mania. The patient returns in 6 weeks with no benefit, and the dosage is raised. She returns 6 weeks later with her husband and is exhibiting symptoms of hypomania with pressured speech, increased activity, and poor sleep. The valproate level is checked and is therapeutic. The sertraline is discontinued, and the patient is started on risperidone due to her level of increased arousal. She and her husband return in 1 week, and her mood and behavior continue to improve. The psychiatrist discusses a referral to a psychologist for trauma-focused psychotherapy. The patient would like to reduce nightmares immediately and asks the psychiatrist if increasing the risperidone dosage would help. This is tried with no benefit and some symptoms of restlessness (akathisia). The patient's mood is stable, and she is tapered off risperidone and placed on prazosin for nightmares. She experiences hypotension during the titration process, and the medication is stopped. She is tried on topiramate for nightmares, which causes some mental clouding but improves the nightmares. Concurrently, the patient receives PE therapy followed by CBT for sleep to address nightmares, and her symptoms resolve. The topiramate is tapered off, and her PTSD symptoms remain improved; her mood is stable with divalproex and lamotrigine for bipolar disorder.

This case illustrates several important issues. No medication is completely safe in pregnancy, so a discussion about conception is part of the pharmacotherapy informed-consent process for women. The comorbid diagnosis of bipolar disorder points toward alternative pharmacotherapies, because the first-line SSRI and SNRI medications may precipitate hypomania or mania. There are no medical comorbidities such as hyperlipidemia or diabetes that might increase the risk of using antipsychotic medication. Here the benefit-to-risk analysis favored the addition of risperidone to the medication regimen. Risperidone is being used appropriately for Bipolar I, although it had no benefit for the patient's PTSD symptoms. Prazosin is helpful in the treatment of nightmares, although some individuals may not tolerate it because of its hypotensive effects. Topiramate is a possible alternative and has been studied in bipolar disorder, although it has not proven effective for mood stabilization (U.S. Department of Veterans Affairs, 2010). Finally, it cannot be overemphasized that evidenced-based, trauma-focused psychotherapy offers a large potential benefit with no medication-related side effects. Fortunately, there was a trained therapist available to provide PE and CBT for sleep to this patient.

CONCLUSION

The atypical antipsychotics and anticonvulsants are off-label treatments for PTSD and may be used effectively for the treatment of comorbid conditions for which they are FDA approved, such as schizophrenia and bipolar disorder, but there is currently not enough evidence to support their use as monotherapy, adjunctive therapy, or first-line treatments for PTSD. Atypical antipsychotics have potential side effects of weight gain, elevations in blood glucose and lipid profiles, and involuntary movement disorders. This requires increased monitoring of lab work, weight, and blood pressure.

In addition, the cost of these medications has been of concern to health systems. A study of VA patients receiving antipsychotic medications concluded that 60.2% were for off-label use, and 40% of these were being used for treatment of PTSD. The clinical indications for and the effects of off-label use were not addressed by the study. It was estimated that in 2007, $4 billion to $5 billion of antipsychotic expenditures for the VA may have been for off-label prescribing (Leslie, Mohamed, & Rosenheck, 2009).

The anticonvulsant studies have demonstrated no benefit for divalproex and tiagabine. Lamotrigine showed benefit in a small placebo-controlled trial. Topiramate has offered the most promising picture in the studies conducted to date. Two of the four studies cited demonstrated statistically significant improvements in total CAPS scores. Of the two remaining studies, one was limited by a high dropout rate, and the other showed statistically significant improvement in the reexperiencing subscale on the CAPS. Topiramate might be considered for refractory patients given the evidence available, but further studies are needed (Andrus & Gilbert, 2010).

The anticonvulsants showing promise in PTSD treatment also have potentially serious side effects. Lamotrigine may cause a severe rash if not titrated properly. Potential side effects of topiramate include cognitive impairment, changes in taste, and overstimulation. Neither of these medications requires routine lab work, however. As with any medication, the potential risks and benefits of the atypical antipsychotics and the anticonvulsants need to be weighed carefully, and the use of evidence-based, trauma-focused psychotherapy must be considered as a first-line choice in PTSD treatment.

REFERENCES

Akuchekian, S., & Amanat, S. (2004). The comparison of topiramate and placebo in the treatment of posttraumatic stress disorder: A randomized, double-blind study. *Journal of Research in Medical Sciences, 5*, 240–244.

Andrus, M. R., & Gilbert, E. (2010). Treatment of civilian and combat-related posttraumatic stress disorder with topiramate. *Annals of Pharmacotherapy, 44*, 1810–1816. doi:10.1345/aph.1P163; 10.1345/aph.1P163

Bartzokis, G., Lu, P. H., Turner, J., Mintz, J., & Saunders, C. S. (2005). Adjunctive risperidone in the treatment of chronic combat-related posttraumatic stress disorder. *Biological Psychiatry, 57*, 474–479. doi:10.1016/j.biopsych.2004.11.039

Butterfield, M. I., Becker, M. E., Connor, K. M., Sutherland, S., Churchill, L. E., & Davidson, J. R. (2001). Olanzapine in the treatment of post-traumatic stress disorder: A pilot study. *International Clinical Psychopharmacology, 16,* 197–203. doi:10.1097/00004850-200107000-00003

Byers, M. G., Allison, K. M., Wendel, C. S., & Lee, J. K. (2010). Prazosin versus quetiapine for nighttime posttraumatic stress disorder symptoms in veterans: An assessment of long-term comparative effectiveness and safety. *Journal of Clinical Psychopharmacology, 30,* 225–229. doi:10.1097/JCP.0b013e3181dac52f; 10.1097/JCP.0b013e3181dac52f

Carey, P., Suliman, S., Ganesan, K., Seedat, S., & Stein, D. J. (2012). Olanzapine monotherapy in posttraumatic stress disorder: Efficacy in a randomized, double-blind, placebo-controlled study. *Human Psychopharmacology, 27,* 386–391. doi:10.1002/hup.2238; 10.1002/hup.2238

Cloitre, M., Stovall-McClough, K. C., Nooner, K., Zorbas, P., Cherry, S., Jackson, C. L., . . . Petkova, E. (2010). Treatment for PTSD related to childhood abuse: A randomized controlled trial. *The American Journal of Psychiatry, 167,* 915–924. doi:10.1176/appi.ajp.2010.09081247

Davidson, J. R., Brady, K., Mellman, T. A., Stein, M. B., & Pollack, M. H. (2007). The efficacy and tolerability of tiagabine in adult patients with post-traumatic stress disorder. *Journal of Clinical Psychopharmacology, 27,* 85–88. doi:10.1097/JCP.0b013e31802e5115

Davis, L. L., Davidson, J. R., Ward, L. C., Bartolucci, A., Bowden, C. L., & Petty, F. (2008). Divalproex in the treatment of posttraumatic stress disorder: A randomized, double-blind, placebo-controlled trial in a veteran population. *Journal of Clinical Psychopharmacology, 28,* 84–88. doi:10.1097/JCP.0b013e318160f83b

Foa, E. B., Keane, T. M., Friedman, M. J., & Cohen, J. A. (Eds.). (2009). *Effective treatments for PTSD: Practice guidelines from the International Society for Traumatic Stress Studies.* New York, NY: Guilford Press.

Hamner, M. B., Faldowski, R. A., Ulmer, H. G., Frueh, B. C., Huber, M. G., & Arana, G. W. (2003). Adjunctive risperidone treatment in post-traumatic stress disorder: A preliminary controlled trial of effects on comorbid psychotic symptoms. *International Clinical Psychopharmacology, 18,* 1–8. doi:10.1097/00004850-200301000-00001

Hertzberg, M. A., Butterfield, M. I., Feldman, M. E., Beckham, J. C., Sutherland, S. M., Connor, K. M., & Davidson, J. R. (1999). A preliminary study of lamotrigine for the treatment of posttraumatic stress disorder. *Biological Psychiatry, 45,* 1226–1229. doi:10.1016/S0006-3223(99)00011-6

Krystal, J. H., Rosenheck, R. A., Cramer, J. A., Vessicchio, J. C., Jones, K. M., Vertrees, J. E. (2011). Adjunctive risperidone treatment for antidepressant-resistant symptoms of chronic military service-related PTSD: A randomized trial. *JAMA, 306,* 493–502. doi:10.1001/jama.2011.1080

Leslie, D. L., Mohamed, S., & Rosenheck, R. A. (2009). Off-label use of antipsychotic medications in the Department of Veterans Affairs health care system. *Psychiatric Services, 60,* 1175–1181. doi:10.1176/appi.ps.60.9.1175

Lindley, S. E., Carlson, E. B., & Hill, K. (2007). A randomized, double-blind, placebo-controlled trial of augmentation topiramate for chronic combat-related posttraumatic stress disorder. *Journal of Clinical Psychopharmacology, 27,* 677–681. doi:10.1097/jcp.0b013e31815a43ee

Monnelly, E. P., Ciraulo, D. A., Knapp, C., & Keane, T. (2003). Low-dose risperidone as adjunctive therapy for irritable aggression in posttraumatic stress disorder. *Journal of Clinical Psychopharmacology, 23,* 193–196. doi:10.1097/00004714-200304000-00012

Monson, C. M., Schnurr, P. P., Resick, P. A., Friedman, M. J., Young-Xu, Y., & Stevens, S. P. (2006). Cognitive processing therapy for veterans with military-related posttraumatic stress disorder. *Journal of Consulting and Clinical Psychology, 74,* 898–907. doi:10.1037/0022-006X.74.5.898

Padala, P. R., Madison, J., Monnahan, M., Marcil, W., Price, P., Ramaswamy, S., & Petty, F. (2006). Risperidone monotherapy for post-traumatic stress disorder related to sexual assault and domestic abuse in women. *International Clinical Psychopharmacology, 21,* 275–280. doi:10.1097/00004850-200609000-00005

Reich, D. B., Winternitz, S., Hennen, J., Watts, T., & Stanculescu, C. (2004). A preliminary study of risperidone in the treatment of posttraumatic stress disorder related to childhood abuse in women. *Journal of Clinical Psychiatry, 65,* 1601–1606. doi:10.4088/JCP.v65n1204

Resick, P. A., Nishith, P., Weaver, T. L., Astin, M. C., & Feuer, C. A. (2002). A comparison of cognitive-processing therapy with prolonged exposure and a waiting condition for the treatment of chronic posttraumatic stress disorder in female rape victims. *Journal of Consulting and Clinical Psychology, 70,* 867–879. doi:10.1037/0022-006X.70.4.867

Rothbaum, B. O., Killeen, T. K., Davidson, J. R., Brady, K. T., Connor, K. M., & Heekin, M. H. (2008). Placebo-controlled trial of risperidone augmentation for selective serotonin reuptake inhibitor-resistant civilian posttraumatic stress disorder. *Journal of Clinical Psychiatry, 69,* 520–525. doi:10.4088/JCP.v69n0402

Schnurr, P. P., Friedman, M. J., Engel, C. C., Foa, E. B., Shea, M. T., Chow, B. K., . . . Bernardy, N. (2007). Cognitive behavioral therapy for posttraumatic stress disorder in women: A randomized controlled trial. *JAMA, 297,* 820–830. doi:10.1001/jama.297.8.820

Schoenfeld, F. B., Deviva, J. C., & Manber, R. (2012). Treatment of sleep disturbances in posttraumatic stress disorder: A review. *Journal of Rehabilitation Research and Development, 49,* 729–752. doi:10.1682/JRRD.2011.09.0164

Stein, M. B., Kline, N. A., & Matloff, J. L. (2002). Adjunctive olanzapine for SSRI-resistant combat-related PTSD: A double-blind, placebo-controlled study. *The American Journal of Psychiatry, 159,* 1777–1779. doi:10.1176/appi.ajp.159.10.1777

Tripathi, A., & Macaluso, M. (2013). Antipsychotics for nonpsychotic illness: Limited evidence suggests possible efficacy based on known receptor binding affinities. *Current Psychiatry, 12,* 23–29.

Tucker, P., Trautman, R. P., Wyatt, D. B., Thompson, J., Wu, S. C., Capece, J. A., & Rosenthal, N. R. (2007). Efficacy and safety of topiramate monotherapy in civilian posttraumatic stress disorder: A randomized, double-blind, placebo-controlled study. *Journal of Clinical Psychiatry, 68,* 201–206. doi:10.4088/JCP.v68n0204

U.S. Department of Veterans Affairs. (2010). *VA clinical practice guideline for management of bipolar disorder.* Washington, DC: Author. Retrieved from http://www.guideline.gov/content.aspx?id=16314

U.S. Department of Veterans Affairs & Department of Defense. (2010). *VA/DoD Clinical Practice Guidelines. Management of post-traumatic stress and acute stress reaction.* Washington, DC: Author. Retrieved from http://www.healthquality.va.gov/guidelines/MH/ptsd

Yeh, M. S., Mari, J. J., Costa, M. C., Andreoli, S. B., Bressan, R. A., & Mello, M. F. (2011). A double-blind randomized controlled trial to study the efficacy of topiramate in a civilian sample of PTSD. *CNS Neuroscience & Therapeutics, 17,* 305–310. doi:10.1111/j.1755-5949.2010.00188.x; 10.1111/j.1755-5949.2010.00188.x

7

Cognitive Behavioral Therapies for PTSD

Tara E. Galovski and Chelsea Gloth

Over the past several decades, research focusing on the development of cognitive behavioral therapies specifically designed to treat posttraumatic stress disorder (PTSD) has proliferated. Derived from a cognitive behavioral theoretical orientation, a number of specific interventions have demonstrated particularly strong empirical support and, subsequently, have been designated as evidence-based interventions. This chapter provides an overview of the fruits of this substantial body of research, with the ultimate goal of providing clinicians guidance in formulating treatment plans for survivors of trauma who suffer from PTSD.

---

http://dx.doi.org/10.1037/14522-008
A Practical Guide to PTSD Treatment: Pharmacological and Psychotherapeutic Approaches,
N. C. Bernardy and M. J. Friedman (Editors)
Copyright © 2015 by the American Psychological Association. All rights reserved.

COGNITIVE BEHAVIORAL THERAPY

The label *cognitive behavioral therapy* (CBT) represents a broad class of individual therapies identified by adherence to several important features. By definition, CBTs are time-limited therapies with specific treatment goals involving the remediation of identified symptoms. Patients and therapists engage in an atmosphere of collaborative empiricism to achieve these therapeutic goals with outcomes evaluated using observable measures of symptom amelioration. Thus, CBTs are amendable to scientific investigation and, in fact, many cognitive behavioral–oriented interventions have enjoyed significant empirical success across a variety of clinical presentations and psychiatric disorders.

Because of the accumulation of empirical support for numerous CBTs, a variety of national and international organizations have begun developing clinical practice guidelines for specific disorders to guide practitioners in navigating the extant literature and to inform clinical care. PTSD is no exception, and numerous organizations have conducted systematic reviews of the trauma intervention literature with the goal of developing best practice guidelines (BPGs). Recently Forbes et al. (2010) published a "guide to guidelines," sorting through the rather extensive collection of published (and, at times, discrepant) BPGs for treating PTSD across national and international organizations. The authors concluded that the various guidelines reviewed all "strongly support the use of trauma-focused psychological treatment in PTSD" (p. 544) and recognized that there is less consensus across published practice guidelines on the relative strength of endorsement of one particular intervention over another. This chapter describes the various CBTs for PTSD that have demonstrated efficacy through the course of randomized clinical trials (RCTs) and includes a brief review of the literature supporting each intervention. We focus primarily on the interventions that have been most widely recognized as BPGs and also recognize those that show promising empirical support. Attention is paid to reductions in important clinical correlates and the use of the interventions in special populations, such as complex trauma and applications with diverse samples.

EVIDENCE-BASED CBTS FOR PTSD

Stress Inoculation Training

Originally developed by Meichenbaum (1974) to treat general manifestations of anxiety, stress inoculation training (SIT) was the first treatment used to specifically target PTSD. SIT is divided into three phases of treatment consisting first of psychoeducation regarding PTSD and the different "channels" of the fear response (emotional, behavioral, physical, and cognitive). The second phase involves acquisition of skills designed to target fear responses across the four channels. The final phase involves the application of these learned skills in daily, anxiety-provoking situations. SIT was used as a comparison condition in two RCTs testing the efficacy of prolonged exposure (PE). The first trial (Foa, Rothbaum, Riggs, & Murdock, 1991) tested the relative efficacy of SIT, PE, a supportive condition and a waitlist control in a sample of 45 female survivors of rape. All three active conditions were significantly superior to the waitlist condition on PTSD, depression, and anxiety, with SIT emerging as superior to PE at posttreatment. Interestingly, PE was superior to SIT at the follow-up assessment. A second trial (Foa et al., 1999) compared SIT alone with PE alone, a combination of PE and SIT, and a waitlist group in a group of 96 female assault survivors. All three active conditions were again superior to the waitlist group. PE alone was superior to SIT and PE+SIT on PTSD, depression, anxiety, and social adjustment, suggesting that the addition of SIT to the PE protocol has no additive benefit in reducing symptoms.

Prolonged Exposure

Foa and Kozak (1986) offered the theory of emotional processing to explain the development and maintenance of PTSD. Emotional processing theory suggests that pathological fear structures exist in our memory and are (in the case of PTSD) easily activated when an individual is confronted with cues reminiscent of the traumatic event. To target and modify these fear structures through emotional processing, PE seeks to activate the fear structure in a safe environment and allow the survivor to incorporate new and corrective information. Foa and Rothbaum (1998) described the original PE protocol as an intervention ranging in length from nine to 12 sessions, each consisting of 90 minutes of therapy. Following a psychoeducation phase, the therapy includes breathing retraining for anxiety management and two types of exposure therapy: in vivo (gradual confrontation of feared stimuli outside of therapy) and imaginal (the patient closes his or her eyes and recalls the event in the present tense with the guidance of the therapist). The therapist and the patient process the emotion generated by the imaginal exposure in session. The patient is asked to listen to the audiotaped imaginal exposure, engage in the in vivo exposure, and practice the breathing techniques on a daily basis.

PE has been compared with a number of interventions, including treatment as usual (TAU) within a sample of 21 physical and sexual assault survivors (Feske, 2008) and with 30 survivors of combat or terror (Nacasch et al., 2011). In both trials, PE was superior to TAU in improving symptoms of PTSD, depression, and measures of anxiety. In a sample of 284 female veterans and active duty service members treated across 12 sites, Schnurr et al. (2007) reported PE to be superior to present-centered therapy (a supportive condition) on measures of PTSD, depression, anxiety, and overall mental health outcomes. In an effort to improve overall outcomes in PE, Foa et al. (2005) assessed the additive benefit of cognitive restructuring (CR) to the PE protocol, hypothesizing that multiple approaches may be more efficacious than a single technique. Results demonstrated that both PE and PE + CR were superior to the waitlist condition but that there was no added benefit of the cognitive restructuring. Rothbaum et al. (2006) found that the addition of PE to a regimen of sertraline indicated participants receiving PE went on to improve significantly more in PTSD severity over the 5 weeks (compared with participants who continued on with sertraline alone), suggesting an augmentation effect for PE, particularly for participants who had only showed a partial response to sertraline.

Cognitive Processing Therapy

Cognitive processing therapy (CPT) is a predominantly cognitive therapy developed by Patricia Resick specifically to treat PTSD and can be conducted in either group or individual format (Resick, Monson, & Chard, 2010). CPT expands on information processing theory with social cognitive theory, recognizing the importance of the meaningfulness of the event in the development and maintenance of PTSD. The protocol originally included 12 sessions during which the therapist provides psychoeducation from a cognitive perspective. Conceptualizing PTSD as a disorder of nonrecovery, CPT then teaches the client to identify inaccurate thoughts and beliefs that may cause one to become "stuck" in recovery from the traumatic event. Inaccurate, trauma-related thoughts and beliefs (e.g., "I was raped because I wore a short skirt") as well as current thoughts regarding self, others, and world (e.g., "All men can't be trusted") are termed *stuck points*. Once these stuck points have been identified, the therapist and client engage in a process of collaborative empiricism, with the therapist relying heavily on Socratic questions to help guide the client to arrive at more accurate alternative thoughts (e.g., "It wasn't the skirt that caused the rape, it was the rapist"). Simultaneously, in engaging with the memory, the client has the opportunity to process natural affect associated with the memory.

In the first RCT testing the relative efficacy of CPT (Resick, Nishith, Weaver, Astin, & Feuer, 2002), CPT was compared with PE and with waitlist with a sample of 171 female rape survivors. Both active conditions were superior to the waitlist on PTSD and depressive symptoms, with CPT and PE being statistically equivalent on both of these primary outcomes. CPT demonstrated an advantage over PE on measures of guilt (Resick et al., 2002) and on reductions in health-related concerns (Galovski, Monson, Bruce, & Resick, 2009). Treatment gains were well maintained over 5 years for both CPT and PE (Resick, Williams, Suvak, Monson, & Gradus, 2012). Following the demonstration of the efficacy of the full CPT treatment package, Resick et al. (2008) conducted a dismantling study with 150 female survivors of interpersonal violence. This study sought to compare the relative efficacy of the full treatment package of CPT to its two theorized active components, the written account (WA) and the cognitive therapy (CT). All three conditions showed significant improvement; however, the CT condition was statistically superior to the WA condition at several points across therapy, whereas CPT fell in between (with no statistical difference compared with either condition). The authors suggested that the CT condition and full CPT are viable treatment options. CPT has also been shown to be significantly superior to a waitlist in 60 military-related PTSD veterans (Monson et al., 2006) and in the self-report of PTSD of 73 female and 13 male military veteran sexual trauma survivors compared with present-centered therapy (Surís, Link-Malcolm, Chard, Ahn, & North, 2013).

Chard (2005) compared CPT for 71 survivors of childhood sexual abuse (CPT–SA; CPT modified to include an additional five sessions in combined group and individual format) to a minimal attention control condition. CPT–SA was significantly more effective at reducing trauma-related symptoms with excellent maintenance over the 1-year follow-up interval. Finally, Galovski, Blain, Mott, Elwood, and Houle (2012) modified the traditional 12-session duration of CPT by allowing patient progress to determine the end of therapy with 100 male and female survivors of interpersonal trauma. Treatment end was determined by good end-state functioning scores on PTSD and depression symptom measures. The CPT condition reported significantly greater improvement on all outcomes compared with the minimal attention condition. Interestingly, 58% of the sample met good end-state functioning before session 12, and 34% required more therapy to meet this end state. At the 3-month follow-up, 48 of 50 (96%) of the study participants had lost their PTSD diagnosis. These results suggest continued benefit of further treatment when necessary. Furthermore, this trial sought to identify sex differences in outcomes in civilian rape and physical assault survivors. Galovski, Blain, Chappuis, and Fletcher (2013) found that men and women respond similarly over a course of CPT with respect to PTSD and depressive symptom reductions. However, women evidenced more rapid gains on measures of guilt, anger and irritability, and dissociation.

Eye Movement Desensitization and Reprocessing

Eye movement desensitization and reprocessing (EMDR) was first developed by Francine Shapiro (1989) as a treatment for traumatic memories and PTSD. EMDR has been a fairly controversial treatment largely because of the lack of theoretical foundation and lack of empirical support for the lateral eye movements contained in the protocol (Spates, Koch, Cusack, Paato, & Waller, 2009), as well as a history of studies with significant methodological limitations. During the intervention, patients are asked to visualize their traumatic event while visually tracking the therapist's finger as it moves back and forth (or some other form of bilateral stimulation). Recently, several trials showed support for the efficacy of EMDR as an exposure therapy, although less support was evidenced for the importance of the eye movement component (reviewed in Forbes et al., 2010).

Imagery Rehearsal Therapy

Imagery rehearsal therapy (IRT) is perhaps most frequently recommended as an additive therapy, used before one of the therapies just described, for cases with profound nightmares or individuals presenting with residual nightmares after a course of PTSD intervention (Moore & Krakow, 2010). IRT can be conducted in either group or individual format and consists of rescripting the narrative of one's nightmares by changing and rehearsing a more desirable outcome. This intervention has been particularly effective in reducing both nightmares and insomnia (Moore & Krakow, 2010) compared with a waitlist control (Krakow et al., 2001) and with a generic sleep and nightmare treatment (Cook et al., 2010).

Finally, a host of studies conducted across trauma samples have used more general cognitive behavioral interventions to treat PTSD. These interventions use a multifaceted treatment approach, including psychoeducation, progressive muscle relaxation, imaginal and in vivo exposure, cognitive restructuring, coping strategies, and other behavioral interventions. Examples of success using these interventions include significant reductions of PTSD symptoms in motor vehicle accident survivors compared with a supportive condition (Blanchard et al., 2003) and with a minimal contact condition (Beck, Coffey, Foy, Keane, & Blanchard, 2009), in survivors of interpersonal assault (McDonagh et al., 2005), and in individuals exposed to combat trauma (Schnurr et al., 2003) when CBT was compared with person-centered therapy. Cognitive therapy has shown similar improvements in PTSD across a range of trauma types compared with waitlist in survivors of terrorism and conflict (Duffy, Gillespie, & Clark, 2007), survivors of motor vehicle accidents (Ehlers et al., 2003), and battered women (Kubany et al., 2004).

Finally, for children and adolescents, trauma-focused cognitive behavioral therapy (TF–CBT) has accumulated the most empirical support in treating PTSD. This treatment model adopts a broad-based approach to target difficulties in a host of domains of functioning, including behavioral, cognitive, affective, and physiological arenas. Importantly, this intervention includes the primary caregiver to assist the adult in coping with the child's distress. Thus, the treatment format includes individual sessions for child and caregiver as well as conjoint sessions. Two large-scale field trials were conducted including children ages 8 to 14 years with results showing significantly greater improvements for TF–CBT compared with client-centered treatment in PTSD, depression, distress, parental support of child, and positive parenting practices (Cohen, Deblinger, & Mannarino, 2005; Cohen, Deblinger, Mannarino, & Steer, 2004).

PHARMACOTHERAPY AND CBTS

Clinical practice guidelines differ on the use of medication as a first-line intervention in treating PTSD. The use of pharmacotherapy as a solitary treatment approach is reviewed in Williams, Richardson, and Galovski (2013). Relatively few RCTs have addressed the question of additive benefits of combination approaches of medication and psychotherapy in treating PTSD. One of the primary considerations in implementing this course of treatment is the temporal administration of the therapies. Rothbaum et al. (2006) added a course of PE to a regimen of sertraline if an improvement of at least 20% in PTSD symptoms was observed after

10 weeks of the pharmacotherapy. The comparison condition continued on with another 5 weeks of sertraline only. Although there was a higher dropout rate for those who received PE, the addition of PE did appear to further reduce PTSD severity (but not depression or anxiety). Contrarily, Schneier and colleagues (2012) first administered 10 sessions of PE to study participants and then randomized participants to either 12 weeks of paroxetine or 12 weeks of placebo. Patients who received paroxetine experienced significantly greater improvements in PTSD. Of specific note, clinical guidelines have suggested that the use of benzodiazepines, other anxiolytics, and sedative hypnotics may, in fact, reduce the efficacy of psychotherapy (particularly exposure-based therapies) and caution the potential for harm (U.S. Department of Veteran Affairs & Department of Defense, 2010; for a review of the use of benzodiazepines with PTSD, see Bernardy, 2013; see also Chapter 5, this volume). Given that a combined approach of medication and psychotherapy is likely common in clinical practice, additional research is warranted looking at combinations of various classes of medications as they interact with various types of cognitive behavioral interventions. Although the empirical support for the use of medications as a first-line treatment is not as strong as that for CBTs (Friedman, Davidson, & Stein, 2009), medications can play an important role in overall outcomes. Combined medication plus CBT may serve to ameliorate symptoms associated with the additional psychiatric disorders that co-occur with PTSD. Finally, medications may certainly play in role in overall outcomes in decreasing non-PTSD symptoms that may interfere with an individual's ability to engage in PTSD psychotherapy (Friedman et al., 2009). In summary, the American Psychiatric Association (Benedek, Friedman, Zatzick, & Ursano, 2009) currently supports the use of selective serotonin reuptake inhibitors and serotonin norepinephrine reuptake inhibitors for the treatment of PTSD.

Investigators have made remarkable progress in developing efficacious interventions for PTSD. CBTs appear to largely result in improvements in symptoms of PTSD and depression. Therapy success transcends the core symptoms of PTSD and is evident in important areas of client functioning even after the completion of treatment, as measured by improvements in general psychosocial functioning in multiple channel exposure therapy (Falsetti, Erwin, Resnick, Davis, & Combs-Lane, 2003) and, specifically, in engagement in leisure activities and social, occupational, interpersonal, and sexual functioning in both CPT and PE (Galovski, Sobel, Phipps, & Resick, 2005). Recent neuroimaging research suggests that CBT influences and improves dysregulated areas in the brain typically associated with PTSD—namely, the amygdala and insula activity (Bryant et al., 2008). Results from recent studies suggest that neural circuitry underlying inhibitory control may be involved in changes in PTSD during CBT (Falconer, Allen, Femingham, Williams, & Bryant, 2013). Additional investigations of the neural bases of response to CBTs will further inform both the interventions themselves and the role of pharmacotherapy in successful outcomes.

Cognitive behavioral interventions continue to be modified and improved through empirical investigation, including modifications of protocols in terms of therapy duration (Chard, 2005; Galovski et al., 2012), additional treatment components (Ironson, Freund, Strauss, & Williams, 2002), augmentation with pharmacotherapy (Rothbaum et al., 2006), in combination with different interventions to treat comorbid conditions (e.g., panic—Falsetti, Resnick, Davis, & Gallagher, 2001; borderline personality—Clarke, Rizvi, & Resick, 2008), and across diverse populations including Bosnian (Schulz, Resick, Huber, & Griffin, 2006) and Vietnamese refugees (Hinton et al., 2004). Although no RCTs examining the efficacy of CBT treatments for PTSD have been conducted specifically in geriatric samples to date, several case studies with geriatric clients have been conducted, and results suggest that cognitive behavioral interventions are effective in older adults (Clapp & Beck, 2012), despite some clinical speculation that CBTs may exacerbate age-related medical conditions or fragility (Hankin, 1997) or may be less effective due to age-related declines in cognitive flexibility or capacity (Flint, 2004).

The plethora of gold standard research trials have resulted in BPGs translating the fruits of academia to actual clinical practice with an eye to the dissemination and implementation of these interventions (Cook, Schnurr, & Foa, 2004). The benefits of such guidelines are exemplified in the historic rollout of these interventions across the Veterans Health Administration (Karlin et al., 2010). Similar rollouts at the state level and in civilian entities must follow. Dissemination of these interventions has also occurred internationally in a number of developing countries. For example, Kaysen et al. (2013) described excellent results in bringing CPT to Iraq, tailoring the intervention to meet the specific needs of this low-resource country including incorporating specific beliefs and structures in the Kurdish culture and accounting for significant language barriers and low literacy rates. All told, the intervention research in the field of trauma recovery has advanced in leaps and bounds. We look forward to what the future holds as we continue to hone and adapt our interventions to best meet the needs of survivors of trauma.

REFERENCES

Beck, J. G., Coffey, S. F., Foy, D. W., Keane, T. M., & Blanchard, E. B. (2009). Group cognitive behavior therapy for chronic posttraumatic stress disorder: An initial randomized pilot study. *Behavior Therapy, 40*, 82–92. doi:10.1016/j.beth.2008.01.003

Benedek, D. M., Friedman, M. J., Zatzick, D., & Ursano, R. J. (2009). Practice guideline for the treatment of patients with acute stress disorder and posttraumatic stress disorder. *Psychiatry Online*. Retrieved from http://www.psychiatryonline.com/content.aspx?aid=156498

Bernardy, N. C. (2013). The role of benzodiazepines in the treatment of posttraumatic stress disorder (PTSD). *PTSD Research Quarterly, 23*, 2–9.

Blanchard, E. B., Hickling, E. J., Devineni, T., Veazey, C. H., Galovski, T. E, Mundy, E., . . . Buckley, T. C. (2003). A controlled evaluation of cognitive behavioural therapy for posttraumatic stress disorder in motor vehicle accident survivors. *Behaviour Research and Therapy, 41*, 79–96. doi:10.1016/S0005-7967(01)00131-0

Bryant, R. A., Felmingham, K., Kemp, A., Das, P., Hughes, G., Peduto, A., & Williams, L. (2008). Amygdala and ventral anterior cingulate activation predicts treatment response to cognitive behavior therapy for posttraumatic stress disorder. *Psychological Medicine, 38*, 555–561. doi:10.1017/S0033291707002231

Chard, K. M. (2005). An evaluation of cognitive processing therapy for the treatment of posttraumatic stress disorder related to childhood sexual abuse. *Journal of Consulting and Clinical Psychology, 73*, 965–971. doi:10.1037/0022-006X.73.5.965

Clapp, J. D., & Beck, J. G. (2012). Treatment of PTSD in older adults: Do cognitive-behavioral interventions remain viable? *Cognitive and Behavioral Practice, 19*, 126–135. doi:10.1016/j.cbpra.2010.10.002

Clarke, S. B., Rizvi, S. L., & Resick, P. A. (2008). Borderline personality characteristics and treatment outcome in cognitive-behavioral treatments for PTSD in female rape victims. *Behavior Therapy, 39*, 72–78. doi:10.1016/j.beth.2007.05.002

Cohen, J. A., Deblinger, E., & Mannarino, A. P. (2005). Trauma-focused, cognitive behavioral therapy for sexually abused children. In E. Hibbs & P. Jensen (Eds.), *Psychosocial treatments for child and adolescent disorders: Empirically based strategies for clinical practice* (2nd ed., pp. 743–765). Washington, DC: American Psychological Association.

Cohen, J. A., Deblinger, E., Mannarino, A. P., & Steer, R. A. (2004). A multisite, randomized controlled trial for sexually abused children with PTSD symptoms. *Journal of the American Academy of Child & Adolescent Psychiatry, 43*, 393–402. doi:10.1097/00004583-200404000-00005

Cook, J. M., Harb, G. C., Gehrman, P. R., Cary, M. S., Gamble, G. M., Forbes, D., & Ross, R. J. (2010). Imagery rehearsal for posttraumatic nightmares: A randomized controlled trial. *Journal of Traumatic Stress, 23*, 553–563. doi:10.1002/jts.20569

Cook, J. M., Schnurr, P. P., & Foa, E. B. (2004). Bridging the gap between posttraumatic stress disorder research and clinical practice: The example of exposure therapy. *Psychotherapy: Theory, Research, Practice, Training, 41*, 374–387. doi:10.1037/0033-3204.41.4.374

Duffy, M., Gillespie, K., & Clark, D. M. (2007). Post-traumatic stress disorder in the context of terrorism and other civil conflict in Northern Ireland: Randomised controlled trial. *BMJ: British Medical Journal, 334*, 1147–1150. doi:10.1136/bmj.39021.846852.BE

Ehlers, A., Clark, D. M., Hackmann, A., McManus, F., Fennell, M., Herbert, C., & Mayou, R. (2003). A randomized controlled trial of cognitive therapy, a self-help booklet, and repeated assessments as early interventions for posttraumatic stress disorder. *Archives of General Psychiatry, 60*, 1024–1032. doi:10.1001/archpsyc.60.10.1024

Falconer, E., Allen, A., Felmingham, K. L., Williams, L. M., & Bryant, R. A. (2013). Inhibitory neural activity predicts response to cognitive-behavioral therapy for posttraumatic stress disorder. *Journal of Clinical Psychiatry, 74*, 895–901. doi:10.4088/JCP.12m08020

Falsetti, S. A., Erwin, B. A., Resnick, H. S., Davis, J., & Combs-Lane, A. M. (2003). Multiple channel exposure therapy of PTSD: Impact of treatment on functioning and resources. *Journal of Cognitive Psychotherapy, 17,* 133–147. doi:10.1891/jcop.17.2.133.57439

Falsetti, S. A., Resnick, H. S., Davis, J., & Gallagher, N. G. (2001). Treatment of posttraumatic stress disorder with comorbid panic attacks: Combining cognitive processing therapy with panic control treatment techniques. *Group Dynamics: Theory, Research & Practice, 5,* 252–260. doi:10.1037/1089-2699.5.4.252

Feske, U. (2008). Treating low-income and minority women with posttraumatic stress disorder: A pilot study comparing prolonged exposure and treatment as usual conducted by community therapists. *Journal of Interpersonal Violence, 23,* 1027–1040. doi:10.1177/0886260507313967

Flint, A. J. (2004). Anxiety disorders. In J. Sadavoy, L. Jarvik, G. Grossberg, & B. Meyers (Eds.), *Comprehensive textbook of geriatric psychiatry* (3rd ed., pp. 678–699). New York, NY: Norton.

Foa, E. B., Dancu, C. V., Hembree, E. A., Jaycox, L. H., Meadows, E. A., & Street, G. P. (1999). A comparison of exposure therapy, stress inoculation training, and their combination for reducing posttraumatic stress disorder in female assault victims. *Journal of Consulting and Clinical Psychology, 67,* 194–200. doi:10.1037/0022-006X.67.2.194

Foa, E. B., Hembree, E. A., Cahill, S. P., Rauch, S. A. M., Riggs, D. S., Feeny, N. C., & Yadin, E. (2005). Randomized trial of prolonged exposure for posttraumatic stress disorder with and without cognitive restructuring: Outcome at academic and community clinics. *Journal of Consulting and Clinical Psychology, 73,* 953–964. doi:10.1037/0022-006X.73.5.953

Foa, E. B., & Kozak, M. J. (1986). Emotional processing of fear: Exposure to corrective information. *Psychological Bulletin, 99,* 20–35. doi:10.1037/0033-2909.99.1.20

Foa, E. B., & Rothbaum, B. O. (1998). *Treating the trauma of rape: Cognitive-behavioral therapy for PTSD.* New York, NY: Guilford Press.

Foa, E. B., Rothbaum, B. O., Riggs, D. S., & Murdock, T. B. (1991). Treatment of posttraumatic stress disorder in rape victims: A comparison between cognitive-behavioral procedures and counseling. *Journal of Consulting and Clinical Psychology, 59,* 715–723. doi:10.1037/0022-006X.59.5.715

Forbes, D., Creamer, M., Bisson, J. I., Cohen, J. A., Crow, B. E., Foa, E. B., . . . Ursano, R. J. (2010). A guide to guidelines for the treatment of PTSD and related conditions. *Journal of Traumatic Stress, 23,* 537–552. doi:10.1002/jts.20565

Friedman, M. J., Davidson, J. R. T., & Stein, D. J. (2009). Psychopharmacology for adults. In E. B. Foa, T. M. Keane, M. J. Friedman, & J. A. Cohen (Eds.), *Effective treatments for PTSD: Practice guidelines from the International Society for Traumatic Stress Studies* (2nd ed., pp. 245–268). New York, NY: Guilford Press.

Galovski, T. E., Blain, L. M., Chappuis, C., & Fletcher, T. (2013). Sex differences in recovery from PTSD in male and female interpersonal assault survivors. *Behaviour Research and Therapy, 51*, 247–255. doi:10.1016/j.brat.2013.02.002

Galovski, T. E., Blain, L. M., Mott, J. M., Elwood, L., & Houle, T. (2012). Manualized therapy for PTSD: Flexing the structure of cognitive processing therapy. *Journal of Consulting and Clinical Psychology, 80*, 968–981. doi:10.1037/a0030600

Galovski, T. E., Monson, C. A., Bruce, S., & Resick, P. A. (2009). Does cognitive-behavioral therapy for PTSD improve perceived health? *Journal of Traumatic Stress, 22*, 197–204. doi:10.1002/jts.20418

Galovski, T. E., Sobel, A. A., Phipps, K. A., & Resick, P. A. (2005). Trauma recovery: Beyond posttraumatic stress disorder and other Axis I symptom severity. In T. A. Corales (Ed.), *Trends in posttraumatic stress disorder research* (pp. 207–227). Hauppauge, NY: Nova Science.

Hankin, C. S. (1997). Treatment of older adults with posttraumatic stress disorder. In A. Maercker (Ed.), *Treatment of PTSD* (pp. 357–384). New York, NY: Springer.

Hinton, D. E., Pham, T., Tran, M., Safren, S. A., Otto, M. W., & Pollack, M. H. (2004). CBT for Vietnamese refugees with treatment-resistant PTSD and panic attacks: A pilot study. *Journal of Traumatic Stress, 17*, 429–433. doi:10.1023/B:JOTS.0000048956.03529.fa

Ironson, G., Freund, B., Strauss, J. L., & Williams, J. (2002). Comparison of two treatments for traumatic stress: A community-based study of EMDR and prolonged exposure. *Journal of Clinical Psychology, 58*, 113–128. doi:10.1002/jclp.1132

Karlin, B. E., Ruzek, J. I., Chard, K. M., Eftekhari, A., Monson, C. M., Hembree, E. A., . . . Foa, E. B. (2010). Dissemination of evidence-based psychological treatments for posttraumatic stress disorder in the Veterans Health Administration. *Journal of Traumatic Stress, 23*, 663–673. doi:10.1002/jts.20588

Kaysen, D., Lindgren, K., Zangana, G. A. S., Murray, L., Bass, J., & Bolton, P. (2013). Adaptation of cognitive processing therapy for treatment of torture victims: Experience in Kurdistan, Iraq. *Psychological Trauma: Theory, Research, Practice, and Policy, 5*, 184–192. doi:10.1037/a0026053

Krakow, B., Hollifield, M., Johnston, L., Koss, M., Schrader, R., Warner, T. D., . . . Prince, H. (2001). Imagery rehearsal therapy for chronic nightmares in sexual assault survivors with posttraumatic stress disorder: A randomized controlled trial. *JAMA, 286*, 537–545. doi:10.1001/jama.286.5.537

Kubany, E. S., Hill, E. E., Owens, J. A., Iannce-Spencer, C., McCraig, M. A., Tremayne, K. J., & Williams, P. L. (2004). Cognitive trauma therapy for battered women with PTSD (CTT–BW). *Journal of Consulting and Clinical Psychology, 72*, 3–18.

McDonagh, A., Friedman, M., McHugo, G., Ford, J., Sengupta, A., Mueser, K., . . . Descamps, M. (2005). Randomized trial of cognitive-behavioral therapy for chronic posttraumatic stress disorder in adult female survivors of childhood sexual abuse. *Journal of Consulting and Clinical Psychology, 73*, 515–524. doi:10.1037/0022-006X.73.3.515

Meichenbaum, D. (1974). Self instructional methods. In F. H. Kanfer & A. P. Goldstein (Eds.), *Helping people change* (pp. 357–391). New York, NY: Pergamon Press.

Monson, C. M., Schnurr, P. P., Resick, P. A., Friedman, M. J., Young-Xu, Y., & Stevens, S. P. (2006). Cognitive processing therapy for veterans with military-related posttraumatic stress disorder. *Journal of Consulting and Clinical Psychology, 74*, 898–907. doi:10.1037/0022-006X.74.5.898

Moore, B. A., & Krakow, B. (2010). Imagery rehearsal therapy: An emerging treatment for posttraumatic nightmares in veterans. *Psychological Trauma: Theory, Research, Practice, and Policy, 2*, 232–238. doi:10.1037/a0019895

Nacasch, N., Foa, E. B., Huppert, J. D., Tzur, D., Fostick, L., Dinstein, Y., . . . Zohar, J. (2011). Prolonged exposure therapy for combat- and terror-related posttraumatic stress disorder: A randomized control comparison with treatment as usual. *Journal of Clinical Psychiatry, 72*, 1174–1180. doi:10.4088/JCP.09m05682blu

Resick, P. A., Galovski, T. E., Uhlmansiek, M. O., Scher, C. D., Clum, G. A., & Young-Xu, Y. (2008). A randomized clinical trial to dismantle components of cognitive processing therapy for posttraumatic stress disorder in female victims of interpersonal violence. *Journal of Consulting and Clinical Psychology, 76*, 243–258. doi:10.1037/0022-006X.76.2.243

Resick, P. A., Monson, P. A., & Chard, K. M. (2010). *Cognitive processing therapy: Veteran/military version*. Washington, DC: Department of Veterans Affairs.

Resick, P. A., Nishith, P., Weaver, T. L., Astin, M. C., & Feuer, C. A. (2002). A comparison of CPT with PE and a waiting condition for the treatment of chronic PTSD in female rape victims. *Journal of Consulting and Clinical Psychology, 70*, 867–879. doi:10.1037/0022-006X.70.4.867

Resick, P. A., Williams, L. F., Suvak, M. K., Monson, C. M., & Gradus, J. L. (2012). Long-term outcomes of cognitive–behavioral treatments for posttraumatic stress disorder among female rape survivors. *Journal of Consulting and Clinical Psychology, 80*, 201–210. doi:10.1037/a0026602

Rothbaum, B. O., Cahill, S. P., Foa, E. B., Davidson, J. R. T., Compton, J., Connor, K., . . . Hahn, C. (2006). Augmentation of sertraline with prolonged exposure in the treatment of posttraumatic stress disorder. *Journal of Traumatic Stress*, *19*, 625–638. doi:10.1002/jts.20170

Schneier, F. R., Neria, Y., Pavlicova, M., Hembree, E. A., Suh, E. J., Amsel, L. V., Marshall, R. D. (2012). Combined prolonged exposure therapy and paroxetine for PTSD related to the World Trade Center attack: A randomized controlled trial. *The American Journal of Psychiatry*, *169*, 80–88.

Schnurr, P. P., Friedman, M. J., Engel, C. C., Foa, E. B., Shea, M. T., Chow, B. K., . . . Bernardy, N. (2007). Cognitive behavioral therapy for posttraumatic stress disorder in women: A randomized controlled trial. *JAMA*, *297*, 820–830. doi:10.1001/jama.297.8.820

Schnurr, P. P., Friedman, M. J., Foy, D. W., Shea, M. T., Hsieh, F. Y., Lavori, P. W., . . . Bernardy, N. C. (2003). Randomized trial of trauma-focused group therapy for posttraumatic stress disorder. *Archives of General Psychiatry*, *60*, 481–489. doi:10.1001/archpsyc.60.5.481

Schulz, P. M., Resick, P. A., Huber, L. C., & Griffin, M. G. (2006). The effectiveness of cognitive processing therapy for PTSD with refugees in a community setting. *Cognitive and Behavioral Practice*, *13*, 322–331. doi:10.1016/j.cbpra.2006.04.011

Shapiro, F. (1989). Eye movement desensitization: A new treatment for posttraumatic stress disorder. *Journal of Behavior Therapy and Experimental Psychiatry*, *20*, 211–217. doi:10.1016/0005-7916(89)90025-6

Spates, R. C., Koch, E., Cusack, K., Paato, S., & Waller, S. (2009). Eye movement desensitization and reprocessing. In E. B. Foa, T. M. Keane, M. J. Friedman, & J. A. Cohen (Eds.), *Effective treatments for PTSD: Practice guidelines from the International Society for Traumatic Stress Studies* (2nd ed., pp. 279–305). New York, NY: Guilford Press.

Surís, A., Link-Malcolm, J., Chard, K., Ahn, C., & North, C. (2013). A randomized clinical trial of cognitive processing therapy for veterans with PTSD related to military sexual trauma. *Journal of Traumatic Stress*, *26*, 28–37. doi:10.1002/jts.21765

U.S. Department of Veteran Affairs & Department of Defense. (2010). *VA/DoD Clinical practice guidelines. Management of posttraumatic stress.* Washington, DC: Author.

Williams, A. M., Richardson, G., & Galovski, T. E. (2013). Posttraumatic stress disorder. In S. M. Stahl & B. A. Moore (Eds.) *Anxiety disorders: A guide for integrating psychopharmacology and psychotherapy* (pp. 176–200). New York, NY: Routledge/Taylor & Francis.

THREE

COMORBID DISORDERS AND UNIQUE PRESENTATIONS

8

PTSD and Insomnia

Jason C. DeViva and Bruce Capehart

Impaired sleep is one of the most common symptoms among individuals diagnosed with posttraumatic stress disorder (PTSD; Ohayon & Shapiro, 2000) and has been described as an "almost universal" complaint in that population (Gellis & Gehrman, 2011). Historically, insomnia (i.e., difficulty initiating and maintaining sleep) has been conceptualized as "part" of PTSD (DeViva, Zayfert, Pigeon, & Mellman, 2005; Harvey, Jones, & Schmidt, 2003; Spoormaker & Montgomery, 2008), and providers often presumed that when PTSD was treated, sleep problems would remit; as a consequence, treatments for PTSD usually do not target sleep specifically (Zayfert & DeViva, 2004).

This view has shifted over time as evidence has indicated a more complex relationship between sleep and posttraumatic stress. Some studies have found that disturbed sleep immediately after a traumatic event is a risk factor for later PTSD (Harvey & Bryant, 1998; Koren, Arnon, Lavie, & Klein, 2002). Other research has suggested that insomnia associated with

http://dx.doi.org/10.1037/14522-009
A Practical Guide to PTSD Treatment: Pharmacological and Psychotherapeutic Approaches,
N. C. Bernardy and M. J. Friedman (Editors)
Copyright © 2015 by the American Psychological Association. All rights reserved.

PTSD can exacerbate other posttraumatic symptoms (Germain, Buysse, & Nofziger, 2008; Krakow et al., 2004; Nishith, Resick, & Mueser, 2001), and many of the common consequences of insomnia, such as irritable mood, poor concentration, negative emotional states, and generally poorer coping skills, are themselves diagnostic criteria for or associated features of PTSD (Harvey et al., 2003; Spoormaker & Montgomery, 2008). Insomnia may also contribute to the medical comorbidity associated with PTSD. Shortened sleep is linked to metabolic changes that can increase risk of weight gain (Van Cauter, Spiegel, Tasali, & Leproult, 2008), and weight gain is a side effect of certain psychiatric medications prescribed for insomnia (Jeffreys, Capehart, & Friedman, 2012). Increased weight is a known risk factor for obstructive sleep apnea, Type II diabetes, the metabolic syndrome, and osteoarthritis. Impaired sleep is associated with increases in coronary artery calcification, a marker for cardiovascular disease (Grandner, Patel, Gehrman, Perlis, & Pack, 2010), which may explain findings that PTSD is an independent determinant of presence and severity of, and mortality from, coronary artery disease (Ahmadi et al., 2011). Ramesh et al. (2012) also found that a 15-day episode of sleep fragmentation was related to decreased visuospatial function, increased anxiety, and increased levels of the pro-inflammatory cytokine tumor necrosis factor (TNF)-alpha in rodents, changes that were attenuated in mice lacking the TNF-alpha gene. In addition, poor sleep associated with PTSD appears to persist after an otherwise positive response to trauma-focused therapy (Zayfert & DeViva, 2004). Taken together, these findings suggest that sleep disturbance is a more central component of PTSD that merits specific assessment and treatment (Harvey et al., 2003; Spoormaker & Montgomery, 2008; Zayfert & DeViva, 2004).

Numerous aspects of PTSD may interact with insomnia. For example, nightmares have been shown to have a strong relationship with difficulty initiating and maintaining sleep in PTSD (DeViva, Zayfert, & Mellman, 2004). Some authors have hypothesized that individuals with PTSD learn to associate nightmares with sleep and therefore may experience increased arousal in the sleep setting or may try to stay awake to avoid distress (Krakow et al., 2000; Neylan et al., 1998). Others have proposed that difficulty initiating and maintaining sleep in PTSD is driven by changes to the arousal system (Harvey et al., 2003). Woodward (1995) noted that sleep is incompatible with the increased arousal necessary for heightened vigilance, and fear of loss of vigilance has been shown to be related to poor sleep quality among combat veterans (Pietrzak, Morgan, & Southwick, 2010). In addition, behavior designed to maintain vigilance or safety at night may interfere with sleep initiation and maintenance (DeViva et al., 2005). Possible biological explanations for the relationship between sleep difficulties and PTSD include the role of the hypothalamic-pituitary-adrenocortical axis and premorbid sleep difficulties. A comparison of subjects with PTSD to trauma-exposed subjects without PTSD and healthy control subjects found that elevated adrenocorticotropic hormone levels were correlated with more nocturnal awakenings, decreased subjective sleep quality, and less time in slow-wave sleep (van Liempt, Arends, & Cluitmans, 2013). Review of the Millennium Cohort Study (Ryan et al., 2007) indicated that among active-duty military personnel who had been deployed during Operation Iraqi Freedom or Operation Enduring Freedom, predeployment sleep of less than 6 hours per night was associated with an elevated risk of a postdeployment diagnosis of PTSD. Among those deployed later in the conflict, sleeping more than 8 hours per night predeployment was also associated with postdeployment PTSD diagnosis (Gehrman et al., 2013). Thus, it is possible that sleep disturbances represent both target symptoms and risk factors in PTSD, the latter being a particularly rich area for ongoing research into the underlying biology of PTSD and identification of persons at risk for developing new-onset PTSD. It also appears that insomnia associated with PTSD has the potential to develop into its own independent syndrome that can persist after other aspects of PTSD have remitted.

The initial step in managing insomnia and PTSD is evaluation for possible aggravating conditions. Sleep can be affected by comorbid psychiatric and medical diagnoses (e.g., mood disorders; chronic pain; medical conditions associated with increased urinary frequency, such as diabetes, prostate hypertrophy, and neurogenic bladder), and primary sleep disorders, such as obstructive sleep apnea, restless legs, or periodic limb movements of sleep. Substance use disorders can disrupt sleep from direct substance effects or substance withdrawal. Traumatic brain injury is associated with both disrupted sleep patterns and an increased prevalence of sleep apnea (Castriotta et al., 2007; Schreiber et al., 2008). Each of these conditions should be considered in the patient with PTSD and insomnia, and if an aggravating condition is suspected, it should be addressed with the appropriate intervention or referral to primary or specialty medical care.

When the diagnosis points to PTSD as the cause for insomnia, the recommended management includes behavior and lifestyle changes, psychotherapy targeted at either PTSD or the specific sleep difficulty, and, if behavior changes and psychotherapy are ineffective or not available, then medication can be considered.

BEHAVIORAL AND LIFESTYLE CHANGES

The initial intervention for insomnia related to PTSD should be behavior change. Recent PTSD treatment guidelines recommend appropriate sleep hygiene habits, reducing or eliminating substances (tobacco, caffeine, and alcohol), and obtaining daily aerobic exercise (U.S. Department of Veterans Affairs & Department of Defense, 2010). Patient education on the relationship of behavior to insomnia can reinforce adherence to recommended behavioral changes. Poor sleep hygiene or evening consumption of nicotine and/or caffeine can lead to initial insomnia. Middle insomnia, on the other hand, is less affected by sleep hygiene but can be aggravated by tobacco or alcohol use. One polysomnogram study of smokers found increased sleep-onset latency and disrupted sleep compared with nonsmokers (Jaehne et al., 2012). Alcohol exerts adverse effects on sleep, including tolerance to the hypnotic effect with several days of continuous use, greater daytime sleepiness after use of alcohol as a sleep aid, and an increased risk of daytime accidents among persons using 1 ounce of alcohol as a nighttime sleep aid (Stein & Friedmann, 2005).

PSYCHOLOGICAL TREATMENTS

There are numerous psychotherapies that target PTSD-related sleep disturbances or factors that may cause or exacerbate those disturbances. Treatment planning should be guided by assessment of trauma history,

PTSD symptoms, sleep habits, beliefs about sleep, nightmares, and other sleep disorders (Schoenfeld, DeViva, & Manber, 2012). Psychological treatments for disturbed sleep associated with PTSD should begin with treating the underlying PTSD. If these interventions are ineffective or not tolerated by the patient, an alternative strategy is to engage the patient in a psychotherapy intended to treat insomnia or nightmares and return later to a PTSD-specific psychotherapy.

Evidence-Based CBT for PTSD

Clinical practice guidelines issued by the Departments of Veterans Affairs and Defense (U.S. Department of Veterans Affairs & Department of Defense, 2010) and the International Society for Traumatic Stress Studies (Foa, Keane, Friedman, & Cohen, 2008) recommend psychotherapy interventions such as evidence-based CBT as first-line treatment options for PTSD. These therapies focus specifically on emotional and cognitive alterations that result from traumatic exposure. The two treatments that have proven most effective are exposure therapy (e.g., Foa, Hembree, & Rothbaum, 2007) and cognitive therapy (e.g., Resick, Monson, & Chard, 2007); both have received the highest levels of recommendation in numerous clinical practice guidelines for PTSD (Forbes et al., 2010). Clinical trials examining these CBT approaches do not comprehensively measure effects on sleep. Those that have indicate that treatment is associated with significant improvements on sleep measures (Galovski, Monson, Bruce, & Resick, 2009; Nishith et al., 2003) and that significant proportions of participants experience remission of sleep problems (Cooper & Clum, 1989; Zayfert & DeViva, 2004).

Eye Movement Desensitization and Reprocessing

Eye movement desensitization and reprocessing (EMDR; Shapiro, 1995) has significant research support for its use with PTSD and is also a first-line treatment in the U.S. Department of Veterans Affairs–Department of Defense (VA/DOD) and International Society for Traumatic Stress Studies clinical practice guidelines (Foa et al., 2008). Despite questions about its mechanism of action (Spates & Koch, 2003) and an overall lack of research looking at the effects of EMDR on sleep, one study found that a small sample of participants with PTSD who received EMDR experienced significant improvements in sleep efficiency and wake time after sleep onset (Raboni, Tufik, & Suchecki, 2006).

Imagery Rehearsal

Originally developed to decrease non–trauma-related nightmares, imagery rehearsal (IR) is a term that comprises numerous imagery-based protocols for reducing trauma-related nightmares. IR protocols typically identify a repetitive distressing nightmare, change a detail of that nightmare, and rehearse the changed version of the nightmare (Gehrman & Harb, 2010). IR received a Level A rating for the treatment of nightmare disorder by the American Academy of Sleep Medicine (Aurora et al., 2010), which further stated that IR "appears to be effective in the management of nightmares exhibited in patients with PTSD as well as idiopathic nightmares" (p. 395). Research generally indicates that IR decreases the frequency and intensity of nightmares, improves sleep, and decreases PTSD symptoms. A recent meta-analysis (Casement & Swanson, 2012) found large effect sizes for nightmare frequency and intensity, sleep, and PTSD symptoms. However, results of studies of IR for PTSD have been inconsistent, and protocols vary widely in their specific instructions (Schoenfeld et al., 2012), explaining why IR was designated a Level C treatment for PTSD in the VA/DoD clinical practice guidelines for PTSD (U.S. Department of Veterans Affairs & Department of Defense, 2010).

CBT for Insomnia

Cognitive behavioral therapy for insomnia (CBT–I) typically includes behavioral (stimulus control, sleep restriction, sleep hygiene) and cognitive techniques (cognitive restructuring) with strong support for stimulus control and sleep restriction as monotherapies (Morin, Culbert, & Schwartz, 1994; Murtagh & Greenwood, 1995). The 2008 practice guideline of the American Academy of Sleep Medicine (Schutte-Rodin, Broch, Buysse, Dorsey, & Sateia, 2008) concluded that CBT–I is "effective and recommended" for the treatment of insomnia and recommended CBT–I in any initial approach to treating insomnia whether the insomnia appears to be an independent condition or related to another medical or psychological condition. To date, only two studies have examined the efficacy of CBT–I alone in the treatment of PTSD-related sleep problems. Both studies found that treatment was associated with significant improvements in sleep but also reported that significant proportions of the small participant samples continued to report sleep problems (DeViva, Zayfert, Pigeon, & Mellman, 2005; Gellis & Gehrman, 2011).

Combined IR and CBT–I

Several studies have combined IR interventions with components of CBT–I and found improved sleep measures (Swanson, Favorite, Horin, & Arnedt, 2009), decreased PTSD symptoms (Davis & Wright, 2007), or both (Ulmer, Edinger, & Calhoun, 2011).

Pharmacological Treatments

The first-line medication for PTSD and insomnia should be a selective serotonin reuptake inhibitor (SSRI) or a selective norepinephrine/serotonin reuptake inhibitor (SNRI) antidepressant to mitigate PTSD symptoms. The effects of antidepressants on sleep disturbances in PTSD were recently reviewed (Nappi, Drummond, & Hall, 2012; Schoenfeld et al., 2012). Overall, SSRI and SNRI antidepressants decrease PTSD symptoms, but there is little evidence to show reduction in insomnia. One study showed improved sleep with nefazodone, an antidepressant with uncommon but potentially serious liver toxicity (Hicks et al., 2002). Trazodone is often prescribed for sleep with little empirical evidence for its use in PTSD. The atypical antipsychotic medications olanzapine and quetiapine were reported effective in a randomized controlled trial (RCT) and retrospective study, respectively, but both medications carry

125

a substantial risk for weight gain and the metabolic syndrome. Benzodiazepines and benzodiazepine receptor agonists are commonly prescribed for PTSD-related sleep disturbances without supporting RCT evidence, and benzodiazepines carry a risk for substance dependence (Nappi et al., 2012; Schoenfeld et al., 2012). However, a 2012 meta-analysis examined all premarketing studies submitted to the U.S. Food and Drug Administration for zolpidem, zaleplon, and eszopiclone and found positive but small effects on sleep latency for the medication after adjusting for the effect of placebo (Huedo-Medina, Kirsch, Middlemass, Klonizakis, & Siriwardena, 2012). Additionally, the placebo response represented approximately half of the overall drug response, leading the authors to recommend careful assessment of risks and benefits of hypnotic medication and further attention to psychological interventions for insomnia (Huedo-Medina et al., 2012). These results agree with a meta-analysis showing a small to medium effect size for pharmacological placebo in 23 RCTs for insomnia interventions (Bélanger et al., 2007).

If an SSRI or SNRI antidepressant creates a lower PTSD symptom burden but nightmares persist, prazosin has been demonstrated to be helpful in several placebo-controlled trials (Raskind et al., 2003, 2007). Prazosin was compared in a placebo-controlled RCT to a cognitive behavioral intervention for sleep, and both active treatments produced clinically meaningful results (Germain et al., 2012). Prazosin was found to be as effective as but better tolerated than quetiapine for sleep problems in a retrospective study of veterans (Byers, Allison, Wendel, & Lee, 2010). Overall, prazosin shows the greatest efficacy in relieving PTSD-related insomnia.

CONCLUSION

Managing sleep difficulties in the patient with PTSD is a considerable clinical challenge. The wise clinician will consider the possibility of a comorbid medical, psychiatric, or substance use disorder that is aggravating PTSD-specific factors in disturbed sleep (see Figure 8.1). Addressing these other conditions may relieve some or most of the clinical complaints,

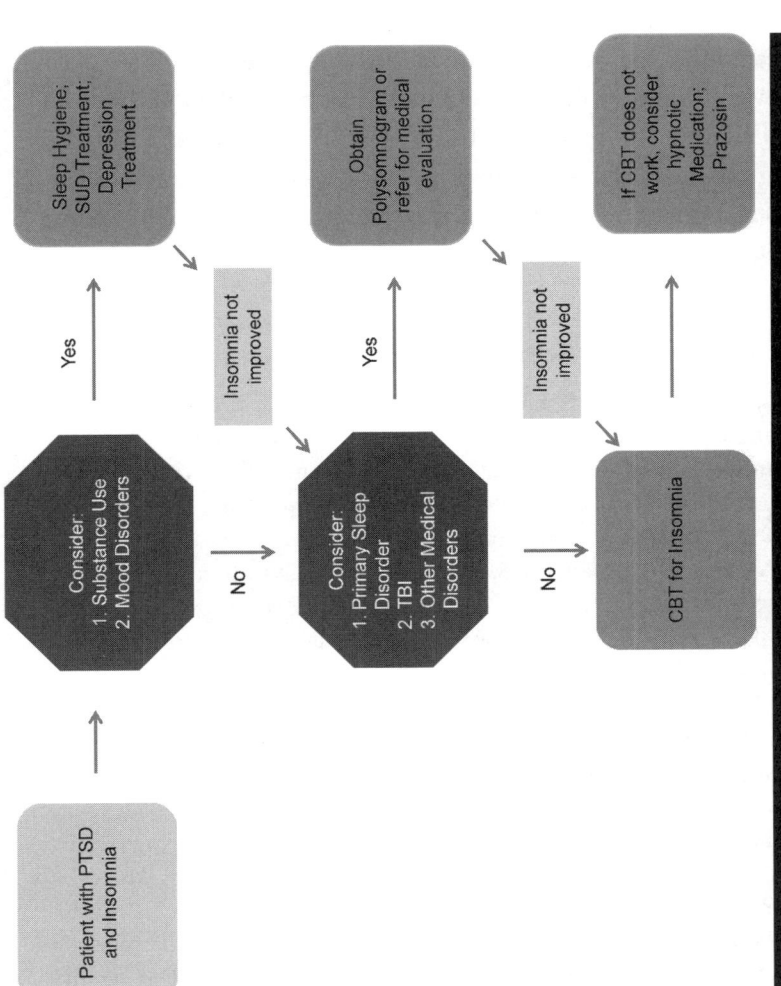

Figure 8.1

Algorithm for assessment and treatment of insomnia associated with posttraumatic stress disorder.
CBT = cognitive behavioral therapy; PTSD = posttraumatic stress disorder; SUD = substance use disorder; TBI = traumatic brain injury.

thereby simplifying treatment and perhaps avoiding another prescription medication. When other aggravating causes are ruled out or adequately addressed, first-line interventions for insomnia include behavior and lifestyle changes, followed by psychotherapies targeted at either trauma or sleep. Medication may contribute to managing sleep difficulties. For most medications, the available clinical evidence does not show clear efficacy, reveals important risk factors that must be weighed in the risk–benefit calculation, or may not clearly separate the pharmacological response from the placebo response. Prazosin appears to be an exception and is recommended for nightmares and disturbed sleep in persons with PTSD.

REFERENCES

Ahmadi, N., Hajsadeghi, F., Blumenthal, R. S., Budoff, M. J., Stone, G. W., & Ebrahimi, R. (2011). Mortality in individuals without known coronary artery disease but with discordance between the Framingham risk score and coronary artery calcium. *The American Journal of Cardiology, 107*, 799–804. doi:10.1016/j.amjcard.2010.10.066

Aurora, R. N., Zak, R. S., Auerbach, S. H., Casey, K. R., Chowdhuri, S., Karippot, A., . . . & Standards of Practice Committee, American Academy of Sleep Medicine (2010). Best practice guide for the treatment of nightmare disorder in adults. *Journal of Clinical Sleep Medicine, 6*, 389–401.

Bélanger, L., Vallieres, A., Ivers, H., Moreau, V., Lavigne, G., & Morin, C. M. (2007). Meta-analysis of sleep changes in control groups of insomnia treatment trials. *Journal of Sleep Research, 16*, 77–84. doi:10.1111/j.1365-2869.2007.00566.x

Byers, M. G., Allison, K. M., Wendel, C. S., & Lee, J. K. (2010). Prazosin versus quetiapine for nighttime posttraumatic stress disorder symptoms in veterans: An assessment of long-term comparative effectiveness and safety. *Journal of Clinical Psychopharmacology, 30*, 225–229. doi:10.1097/JCP.0b013e3181dac52f

Casement, M. D., & Swanson, L. M. (2012). A meta-analysis of imagery rehearsal for post-trauma nightmares: Effects on nightmare frequency, sleep quality, and posttraumatic stress. *Clinical Psychology Review, 32*, 566–574. doi:10.1016/j.cpr.2012.06.002

Castriotta, R., Wilde, M., Lai, J., Atanasov, S., Masel, B., & Kuna, S. (2007). Prevalence and consequences of sleep disorders in traumatic brain injury. *Journal of Clinical Sleep Medicine, 3*, 349–356.

Cooper, N. A., & Clum, G. A. (1989). Imaginal flooding as a supplementary treatment for PTSD in combat veterans: A controlled study. *Behavior Therapy, 20,* 381–391. doi:10.1016/S0005-7894(89)80057-7

Davis, J. L., & Wright, D. C. (2007). Randomized clinical trial for treatment of chronic nightmares in trauma-exposed adults. *Journal of Traumatic Stress, 20,* 123–133. doi:10.1002/jts.20199

DeViva, J. C., Zayfert, C., & Mellman, T. A. (2004). Factors associated with insomnia among civilians seeking treatment for PTSD: An exploratory study. *Behavioral Sleep Medicine, 2,* 162–176. doi:10.1207/s15402010bsm0203_5

DeViva, J. C., Zayfert, C., Pigeon, W. R., & Mellman, T. A. (2005). Treatment of residual insomnia after CBT for PTSD: Case studies. *Journal of Traumatic Stress, 18,* 155–159. doi:10.1002/jts.20015

Foa, E. B., Hembree, E. A., & Rothbaum, B. O. (2007). *Prolonged exposure therapy for PTSD: emotional processing of traumatic experiences: Therapist guide.* New York, NY: Oxford University Press.

Foa, E. B., Keane, T. M., Friedman, M. J., & Cohen, J. A. (Eds.). (2008). *Effective treatments for PTSD: Practice guidelines from the International Society for Traumatic Stress Studies* (2nd ed.). New York, NY: Guilford Press.

Forbes, D., Creamer, M., Bisson, J. I., Cohen, J. A., Crow, B. E., Foa, E. B., . . . Ursano, R. J. (2010). A guide to guidelines for the treatment of PTSD and related conditions. *Journal of Traumatic Stress, 23,* 537–552. doi:10.1002/jts.20565

Galovski, T. E., Monson, C., Bruce, S. E., & Resick, P. A. (2009). Does cognitive-behavioral therapy for PTSD improve perceived health and sleep impairment? *Journal of Traumatic Stress, 22,* 197–204. doi:10.1002/jts.20418

Gehrman, P., Seelig, A. D., Jacobson, I. G., Boyko, E. J., Hooper, T. I., Gackstetter, G. D., . . . Smith, T. C. (2013). Predeployment sleep duration and insomnia symptoms as risk factors for new-onset mental health disorders following military deployment. *Sleep: Journal of Sleep and Sleep Disorders Research, 36,* 1009–1018. doi:10.5665/sleep.2798

Gehrman, P. R., & Harb, G. C. (2010). Treatment of nightmares in the context of posttraumatic stress disorder. *Journal of Clinical Psychology, 66,* 1185–1194. doi:10.1002/jclp.20730

Gellis, L. A., & Gehrman, P. R. (2011). Cognitive behavioral treatment for insomnia in veterans with long-standing posttraumatic stress disorder: A pilot study. *Journal of Aggression, Maltreatment & Trauma, 20,* 904–916. doi:10.1080/10926771.2011.613448

Germain, A., Buysse, D. J., & Nofziger, E. (2008). Sleep-specific mechanisms underlying posttraumatic stress disorder: integrative review and neurobiological hypotheses. *Sleep Medicine Reviews, 12,* 185–195.

Germain, A., Richardson, R., Moul, D. E., Mammen, O., Haas, G., Forman, S. D., . . . Nofziger, E. A. (2012). Placebo-controlled comparison of prazosin and cognitive-behavioral treatments for sleep disturbances in US military veterans. *Journal of Psychosomatic Research, 72*, 89–96. doi:10.1016/j.jpsychores.2011.11.010

Grandner, M. A., Patel, N. P., Gehrman, P. R., Perlis, M. L., & Pack, A. I. (2010). Problems associated with short sleep: Bridging the gap between laboratory and epidemiological studies. *Sleep Medicine Reviews, 14*, 239–247. doi:10.1016/j.smrv.2009.08.001

Harvey, A. G., & Bryant, R. A. (1998). The relationship between acute stress disorder and posttraumatic stress disorder: A prospective evaluation of motor vehicle accident survivors. *Journal of Consulting and Clinical Psychology, 66*, 507–512.

Harvey, A. G., Jones, C., & Schmidt, D. A. (2003). Sleep and posttraumatic stress disorder: A review. *Clinical Psychology Review, 23*, 377–407.

Hicks, J. A., Argyropoulos, S. V., Rich, A. S., Nash, J., Bell, C. J., Edwards, C., . . . Wilson, S. J. (2002). Randomised controlled study of sleep after nefazodone or paroxetine treatment in out-patients with depression. *British Journal of Psychiatry, 180*, 528–535. doi:10.1192/bjp.180.6.528

Huedo-Medina, T. B., Kirsch, I., Middlemass, J., Klonizakis, M., & Siriwardena, A. N. (2012). Effectiveness of non-benzodiazepine hypnotics in treatment of adult insomnia: Meta-analysis of data submitted to the Food and Drug Administration. *BMJ: British Medical Journal, 345*, e8343. doi:10.1136/bmj.e8343

Jaehne, A., Unbehaun, T., Feige, B., Lutz, U. C., Batra, A., & Riemann, D. (2012). How smoking affects sleep: A polysomnographical analysis. *Sleep Medicine, 13*, 1286–1292. doi:10.1016/j.sleep.2012.06.026

Jeffreys, M., Capehart, B., & Friedman, M. J. (2012). Pharmacotherapy for posttraumatic stress disorder: Review with clinical applications. *Journal of Rehabilitation Research and Development, 49*, 703–715. doi:10.1682/JRRD.2011.09.0183

Koren, D., Arnon, I., Lavie, P., & Klein, E. (2002). Sleep complaints as early predictors of posttraumatic stress disorder: A 1-year prospective study of injured survivors of motor vehicle accidents. *The American Journal of Psychiatry, 159*, 855–857.

Krakow, B., Haynes, P. L., Warner, T. D., Santana, E. M., Melendrez, D., Warner, T. D., . . . Shafer, L. (2004). Nightmares, insomnia, and sleep disordered breathing in fire evacuees seeking treatment for posttraumatic sleep disturbance. *Journal of Traumatic Stress, 17*, 257–268.

Krakow, B., Hollifield, M., Schrader, R., Koss, M., Tandberg, D., Lauriello, J., . . . Kelner, R. (2000). A controlled study of imagery rehearsal for chronic nightmares in sexual assault survivors with PTSD: A preliminary report. *Journal of Traumatic Stress, 13,* 589–609.

Morin, C. M., Culbert, J. P., & Schwartz, S. M. (1994). Nonpharmacological interventions for insomnia: A meta-analysis of treatment efficacy. *The American Journal of Psychiatry, 151,* 1172–1180.

Murtagh, D. R., & Greenwood, K. M. (1995). Identifying effective psychological treatments for insomnia: A meta-analysis. *Journal of Consulting and Clinical Psychology, 63,* 79–89. doi:10.1037/0022-006X.63.1.79

Nappi, C. M., Drummond, S. P., & Hall, J. M. (2012). Treating nightmares and insomnia in posttraumatic stress disorder: A review of current evidence. *Neuropharmacology, 62,* 576–585. doi:10.1016/j.neuropharm.2011.02.029

Neylan, T. C., Marmar, C. R., Metzler, T. J., Weiss, D. S., Zatzick, D. F., Delucchi, K. L., . . . Schoenfeld, F. B. (1998). Sleep disturbance in the Vietnam generation: Findings from a nationally representative sample of male Vietnam veterans. *The American Journal of Psychiatry, 154,* 1412–1416.

Nishith, P., Duntley, S. P., Domitrovich, P. P., Uhles, M. L., Cook, B. J., & Stein, P. K. (2003). Effect of cognitive behavioral therapy on heart rate variability during REM sleep in female rape victims with PTSD. *Journal of Traumatic Stress, 16,* 247–250. doi:10.1023/A:1023791906879

Nishith, P., Resick, P. A., & Mueser, K. (2001). Sleep difficulties and alcohol use motives in female rape victims with posttraumatic stress disorder. *Journal of Traumatic Stress, 14,* 469–479.

Ohayon, M. M., & Shapiro, C. M. (2000). Sleep disturbances and psychiatric disorders associated with posttraumatic stress disorder in the general population. *Comprehensive Psychiatry, 41,* 469–478. doi:10.1053/comp.2000.16568

Pietrzak, R. H., Morgan, C. A., & Southwick, S. M. (2010). Sleep quality in treatment-seeking veterans of Operations Enduring Freedom and Iraqi Freedom: The role of cognitive coping strategies and unit cohesion. *Journal of Psychosomatic Research, 69,* 441–448.

Raboni, M. R., Tufik, S., & Suchecki, D. (2006). Treatment of PTSD by eye movement desensitization reprocessing (EMDR) improves sleep quality, quality of life, and perception of stress. *Annals of the New York Academy of Sciences, 1071,* 508–513. doi:10.1196/annals.1364.054

Ramesh, V., Nair, D., Zhang, S. X. L., Hakim, F., Kaushal, N., Kayali, F., . . . Gozal, D. (2012). Disrupted sleep without sleep curtailment induces sleepiness and cognitive dysfunction via the tumor necrosis factor-alpha pathway. *Journal of Neuroinflammation, 9,* 91. doi:10.1186/1742-2094-9-91

Raskind, M. A., Peskind, E. R., Hoff, D. J., Hart, K. L., Holmes, H. A., Warren, D., . . . McFall, M. E. (2007). A parallel group placebo controlled study of prazosin for trauma nightmares and sleep disturbance in combat veterans with post-traumatic stress disorder. *Biological Psychiatry, 61*, 928–934. doi:10.1016/j.biopsych.2006.06.032

Raskind, M. A., Peskind, E. R., Kanter, E. D., Petrie, E. C., Radant, A., Thompson, C. E., . . . McFall, M. M. (2003). Reduction of nightmares and other PTSD symptoms in combat veterans by prazosin: A placebo-controlled study. *The American Journal of Psychiatry, 160*, 371–373. doi:10.1176/appi.ajp.160.2.371

Resick, P. A., Monson, C. M., & Chard, K. M. (2007). *Cognitive processing therapy: Veteran/military version*. Washington, DC: Department of Veterans Affairs.

Ryan, M. A., Smith, T. C., Smith, B., Amoroso, P., Boyko, E. J., Gray, G. C., . . . Hooper, T. I. (2007). Millennium Cohort: Enrollment begins a 21-year contribution to understanding the impact of military service. *Journal of Clinical Epidemiology, 60*, 181–191.

Schoenfeld, F. B., DeViva, J. C., & Manber, R. (2012). Treatment of sleep disturbances in posttraumatic stress disorder: A review. *Journal of Rehabilitation Research and Development, 49*, 729–752. doi:10.1682/JRRD.2011.09.0164

Schreiber, S., Barkai, G., Gur-Hartman, T., Peles, E., Tov, N., Dolberg, O. T., & Pick, C. G. (2008). Long-lasting sleep patterns of adult patients with minor traumatic brain injury (mTBI) and non-mTBI subjects. *Sleep Medicine, 9*, 481–487. doi:10.1016/j.sleep.2007.04.014

Schutte-Rodin, S., Broch, L., Buysse, D., Dorsey, C., & Sateia, M. (2008). Clinical guideline for the evaluation and management of chronic insomnia in adults. *Journal of Clinical Sleep Medicine, 4*, 487–504.

Shapiro, F. (1995). *Eye movement desensitization and reprocessing: Basic principles, protocols, and procedures*. New York, NY: Guilford Press.

Spates, C. R., & Koch, E. I. (2003). From eye movement desensitization and reprocessing to exposure therapy: A review of the evidence for shared mechanisms. *Japanese Journal of Behavior Analysis, 18*, 62–76.

Spoormaker, V. I., & Montgomery, P. (2008). Disturbed sleep in post-traumatic stress disorder: Secondary symptom or core feature? *Sleep Medicine Reviews, 12*, 169–184.

Stein, M. D., & Friedmann, P. D. (2005). Disturbed sleep and its relationship to alcohol use. *Substance Abuse, 26*, 1–13. doi:10.1300/J465v26n01_01

Swanson, L. M., Favorite, T. K., Horin, E., & Arnedt, J. T. (2009). A combined group treatment for nightmares and insomnia in combat veterans: A pilot study. *Journal of Traumatic Stress, 22*, 639–642.

Ulmer, C. S., Edinger, J. D., & Calhoun, P. S. (2011). A multi-component cognitive-behavioral intervention for sleep disturbance in veterans with PTSD: A pilot study. *Journal of Clinical Sleep Medicine, 7,* 57–68.

U.S. Department of Veterans Affairs & Department of Defense. (2010). *Management of post-traumatic stress.* Retrieved from http://www.healthquality.va.gov/Post_Traumatic_Stress_Disorder_PTSD.asp

Van Cauter, E., Spiegel, K., Tasali, E., & Leproult, R. (2008). Metabolic consequences of sleep and sleep loss. *Sleep Medicine, 9*(Suppl. 1), S23–S28. doi:10.1016/S1389-9457(08)70013-3

van Liempt, S., Arends, J., Cluitmans, P. J. M., Westenberg, Kahn, R. S., & Vermetten E. (2013). Sympathetic activity and hypothalomo-pituitary-adrenal axis activity during sleep in post-traumatic stress disorder: A study assessing polysomnography with simultaneous blood sampling. *Psychoneuroendocrinology, 38,* 155–165. doi:10.1016/j.psyneuen.2012.05.015

Woodward, S. (1995). Neurobiological perspectives on sleep in posttraumatic stress disorder. In M. J. Friedman, D. S. Charney, & A. Y. Deutch (Eds.), *Neurobiological and clinical consequences of stress: From normal adaptation to PTSD* (pp. 315–333). Philadelphia, PA: Lippincott-Raven.

Zayfert, C., & DeViva, J. C. (2004). Residual insomnia following cognitive behavioral therapy for PTSD. *Journal of Traumatic Stress, 17,* 69–73. doi:10.1023/B:JOTS.0000014679.31799.e7

9

Co-Occurring Substance Use Disorders and PTSD

Andrew J. Saxon and Tracy L. Simpson

Posttraumatic stress disorder (PTSD) and substance use disorders (SUDs) frequently co-occur (Kessler, Sonnega, Bromet, Hughes, & Nelson, 1995). When the two do co-occur, considerable psychopathologic interplay typically emerges, suggesting the need for treatment of both disorders; however, only a sparse evidence base exists to guide optimal psychopharmacologic or psychotherapeutic treatment for patients with both PTSD and SUD. This chapter reviews the available evidence on treatment of SUD in the presence of PTSD (Berenz & Coffey, 2012; Petrakis et al., 2006; Riggs & Foa, 2008), mentions SUD-specific treatments that clinical experience suggests should be provided to patients with both disorders even if not yet well studied, and speculates on some interventions that

This chapter was coauthored by an employee of the United States government as part of official duty and is considered to be in the public domain. Any views expressed herein do not necessarily represent the views of the United States government, and the author's participation in the work is not meant to serve as an official endorsement.

http://dx.doi.org/10.1037/14522-010
A Practical Guide to PTSD Treatment: Pharmacological and Psychotherapeutic Approaches,
N. C. Bernardy and M. J. Friedman (Editors)
Copyright © 2015 by the American Psychological Association. All rights reserved.

might serve to treat both disorders simultaneously (Kaysen et al., 2014; Raskind et al., 2007; Simpson et al., 2009; Yeh et al., 2011). Some aspects of these topics were recently reviewed in detail (Norman et al., 2012).

DIAGNOSIS

Diagnosis of SUD in patients with PTSD ultimately relies on clinical assessment using *Diagnostic and Statistical Manual of Mental Disorders* (*DSM;* American Psychiatric Association, 2013) or *International Classification of Disease* (*ICD*) criteria. Attempts have been made to align the *DSM* and *ICD* criteria, and, although they are quite similar, they are not identical. Whichever system is used, the criteria for making the diagnosis of SUD are the same across all substances. Regardless of which substance has caused the problem, by the time an individual has developed a diagnosable SUD, the substance use has adversely affected the person's overall level of functioning and his or her physical and mental health and often caused physiologic destabilization.

Screening instruments exist that can help uncover or point the way toward a potential diagnosis. It is important to recognize that a positive screen does not constitute a diagnosis. When individuals screen positive, the screen should be followed up with a complete clinical assessment using the *DSM* or *ICD* criteria to determine if an SUD is present. For alcohol use disorders (AUDs), the Alcohol Use Disorders Identification Test (AUDIT) and the AUDIT—Consumption have been widely validated as self-report screening measures (Bradley et al., 2007; D. M. Donovan, Kivlahan, Doyle, Longabaugh, & Greenfield, 2006). A one-item screening measure was recently validated for drug use disorders consisting of the single question, "How many times in the past year have you used an illegal drug or used a prescription medication for nonmedical reasons?" A response of one time or greater yields a positive screen (Smith, Schmidt, Allensworth-Davies, & Saitz, 2010). In diagnosing PTSD, it is important to be aware that several PTSD symptoms, most notably those in the arousal and reactivity cluster, overlap appreciably with common alcohol withdrawal symptoms (Saladin, Brady, Dansky, & Kilpatrick, 1995) and so care should be taken to ascertain whether these symptoms are present when withdrawal is not occurring.

Treatment of SUD saves lives. For example, tobacco use (primarily smoking) is the number one cause of preventable death resulting in one in four deaths in the United States, mainly from cancers, respiratory disease, and cardiovascular disease (Jha et al., 2013). Excessive alcohol use is the fourth leading cause of death, resulting in an estimated 88,000 deaths and 2.5 million potential years of life lost annually in the United States alone, typically from liver disease, cancers, and cardiovascular disease (Gonzales et al., 2014). Drug overdoses now cause more deaths annually than do motor vehicle accidents (Centers for Disease Control and Prevention, 2014). SUD co-occurring with other psychiatric disorders including PTSD is common and often worsens the course of those other disorders (Blanco et al., 2013; Green, Drake, Brunette, & Noordsy, 2007) and is associated with higher risk for suicide (Schneider, 2009).

TREATMENT STRATEGY

Once a diagnosis is made, the psychopharmacologic and psychotherapeutic management of various SUDs sit on a continuum in which each form of treatment has relatively more or less importance. In the treatment of cannabis and stimulant (cocaine and amphetamines) use disorders, no Food and Drug Administration (FDA)-approved pharmacotherapies exist, and although numerous investigations are seeking effective agents, the mainstay of treatment is psychotherapy. For AUD, the FDA has approved three medications—naltrexone, disulfiram, and acamprosate; topiramate, although not approved, has some demonstrated efficacy. However, for most patients, these medications have only modest efficacy and act as an adjunct to a foundation of psychotherapeutic intervention. For tobacco use disorders (primarily cigarette smoking), medications and psychotherapy both double the odds of quitting and may have additive effects, and both should be used. Opioid use disorders respond exceedingly poorly to behavioral interventions in the absence of medications, so pharmacotherapy is the key treatment component with behavioral interventions as an adjunct.

ALCOHOL USE DISORDERS

Turning first to the pharmacotherapies for AUD, alcohol mobilizes endogenous opioids in the brain, which likely contribute to its euphoric effects (Mitchell et al., 2012). Naltrexone via its antagonism of the mu-opioid receptor putatively makes alcohol less desirable by blocking this euphoria. Naltrexone comes in both an oral formulation and an extended-release intramuscular injection that has activity over a 300-day interval and obviates concerns over adherence to daily oral medication. Disulfiram inhibits the enzyme aldehyde dehydrogenase, a key enzyme in the metabolic pathway for alcohol, thereby causing a buildup of acetaldehyde that results in the unpleasant alcohol-disulfiram reaction if an individual consumes alcohol. Acamprosate and topiramate are proposed to exert their effects by stabilizing inhibitory and excitatory networks in the brain that may be dysregulated by prolonged alcohol use. Both naltrexone and disulfiram reduce alcohol use compared with placebo in veterans with PTSD and AUD without causing any adverse effects on PTSD symptoms but also not exhibiting any particular benefit for PTSD (Petrakis et al., 2006). Acamprosate has not been studied among individuals with co-occurring PTSD and AUD. Although not yet examined in individuals with both disorders, topiramate did demonstrate efficacy for civilian PTSD in a double-blind, placebo controlled trial (Yeh et al., 2011) and thus warrants further study in individuals with co-occurring PTSD and AUD.

TOBACCO USE DISORDERS

Moving to pharmacotherapies for tobacco use disorder, five forms of nicotine replacement therapy (NRT) are FDA approved, with three forms—patch, gum, and lozenge—available over the counter. The nicotine patch comes in three dosage strengths, 21 mg, 14 mg, and 7 mg, which all have a 24-hour duration of action. Most regular tobacco users are started on 21 mg, which supplies roughly the equivalent of the nicotine in a pack of cigarettes, and then use the lower dosage forms to taper off nicotine once abstinence from tobacco is well established. Lighter users of tobacco could potentially start treatment with the lower dosage forms. The gum and lozenge each come in 2- and 4-mg formulations. The 2-mg formulation is for smokers who smoke their first cigarette of the day more than 30 minutes after awakening, and the 4 mg is for smokers who smoke their first cigarette within 30 minutes of awakening. These products can be used every 1 to 2 hours with gradual reduction in dosage after tobacco abstinence is achieved. The nicotine inhaler is a device that allows the user to puff and deliver a dose of nicotine to the oral mucosa from whence it is absorbed. The inhaled nicotine does not go into the lungs. Cartridges each containing 4 mg of nicotine (of which only 2 mg is absorbed) are placed in the device until each cartridge is used up after about 80 inhalations. Individuals quitting can use six to 16 cartridges per day with gradual reduction in dosage once tobacco abstinence is achieved. Nicotine nasal spray delivers about 0.5 mg of nicotine per spray. The user delivers one spray to each nostril every 1 to 2 hours or even more frequently with a maximum of 80 sprays per day; dosage is then gradually reduced once tobacco abstinence is achieved. Nicotine replacement that combines both long-acting and as needed formulations (e.g., patch plus gum or lozenge) is strongly recommended as a first-line approach because the combination has superior efficacy to either alone without any added safety concerns (Fiore, Jaén, & Baker, 2008), and use in hundreds of veterans with PTSD did not indicate any tolerability issues specific to PTSD (McFall et al., 2010).

Bupropion is an antidepressant that purportedly blocks the reuptake of the neurotransmitters dopamine and norepinephrine from the synapse and has antagonist properties at nicotinic receptors. It was evaluated in a small, double-blind, placebo-controlled trial for smoking cessation in veterans with PTSD with some promising evidence for efficacy and no evidence for serious adverse events (Hertzberg, Moore, Feldman, & Beckham, 2001). Varenicline, the most efficacious approved smoking cessation pharmacotherapy (Fiore et al., 2008), is a partial agonist at the alpha4-beta2-nicotinic receptor that mimics some of the reinforcing activity of nicotine while simultaneously blocking nicotine's access to the receptor. Varenicline has an FDA-required boxed warning for psychiatric side effects, although rigorous investigations indicate that, except for sleep disturbance and abnormal dreams, varenicline does not have an elevated psychiatric risk profile above other tobacco-cessation medications or placebo (Garza, Murphy, Tseng, Riordan, & Chatterjee, 2011). Nevertheless, because sleep disturbance and nightmares are hallmarks of PTSD and a retrospective chart review suggested an increase in psychiatric symptomatology among veterans with PTSD treated with varenicline (Campbell & Anderson, 2010), varenicline should be used with close monitoring in individuals with PTSD.

OPIOID USE DISORDERS

Approved pharmacotherapies for opioid use disorders include methadone, buprenorphine, and naltrexone. Methadone acts as a full agonist at the mu-opioid receptor and stimulates it, thus replacing the opioids that were misused. In the United States, methadone can only be provided through federally licensed and accredited opioid treatment programs and is dispensed daily under observation during the initial stages of treatment, which offers often-needed structure but does impose lifestyle limitations. In a randomized controlled trial, methadone, compared with psychosocial intervention without medication, was significantly better at reducing illicit opioid use, keeping patients in treatment, and reducing mortality over a 2-year period (Gunne & Gronbladh, 1981). Preliminary studies suggest that methadone maintenance is effective in treating opioid use disorder among individuals with PTSD (Himelhoch et al., 2012).

Buprenorphine is a partial mu-opioid agonist that also binds to the opioid receptor but does not activate it to the same degree as does a full agonist such as methadone, yet still serves to replace the misused opioids. Because of the lower degree of activation, the risk of a fatal overdose on buprenorphine alone is vanishingly small compared with that risk with full agonist opioids. For that reason, buprenorphine can be prescribed by appropriately trained physicians for patients to obtain at a pharmacy and self-administer. In a randomized controlled trial, buprenorphine maintained patients in treatment significantly longer and reduced mortality in a 1-year period compared with placebo (Kakko, Svanborg, Kreek, &

Heilig, 2003). In the United States, buprenorphine is usually prescribed for opioid use disorder as a sublingual formulation in combination with the opioid antagonist naloxone. Naloxone has poor bioavailability by the sublingual route but discourages misuse by injection because anyone intending to dissolve and inject the sublingual preparation would be injecting an antagonist. Buprenorphine has not been specifically studied in individuals with PTSD.

Naltrexone, as noted, is an opioid antagonist. Before receiving it for an opioid use disorder, patients must be fully withdrawn from opioids, a process that may take 3 to 10 days. Once a patient is on naltrexone, any effects of opioids are totally blocked. Oral naltrexone has not worked well for most patients with opioid use disorder because they tend to discontinue taking it. This problem may be circumvented by use of the long-acting injection form (Krupitsky et al., 2011), but it has not yet been fully investigated in the United States or among individuals with co-occurring PTSD and opioid use disorder.

PSYCHOTHERAPY

Psychotherapy interventions for co-occurring PTSD and SUD have only relatively recently begun to be evaluated. A pressing, but still unanswered, question in the field is whether the two disorders should be treated in an integrated, concurrent fashion or sequentially with the SUD component stabilized before engagement in treatment for the PTSD. Most of the psychotherapy research in this area has focused on the evaluation of various integrated treatments (e.g., B. Donovan, Padin-Rivera, & Kowaliw, 2001; Mills et al., 2012; Najavits et al., 2007; Triffleman, Carroll, & Kellogg, 1999), and to our knowledge sequenced care has not yet been formally evaluated. However, several studies have compared integrated treatments with standard cognitive behavioral (CBT) SUD treatments, and so it is possible to tentatively address the question of whether integrated treatment confers benefit beyond that derived from addressing the SUD.

This literature was recently reviewed by four research teams (Berenz & Coffey, 2012; McCauley, Killeen, Gros, Brady, & Back, 2012; Torchalla,

Nosen, Rostam, & Allen, 2012; van Dam, Vedel, Ehring, & Emmelkamp, 2012). Torchalla et al. (2012) conducted a meta-analysis on the 17 available treatment outcome studies, nine of which were randomized clinical trials. Their within-subject results, which included only patients who received an integrated treatment for PTSD and SUD and compared baseline values with the longest available follow-up assessment, indicated that there was a medium overall effect size for SUD outcomes and a large effect size for PTSD outcomes. However, the between-subjects results involving only those studies that included a control condition, which typically consisted of an SUD-only treatment, did not find a reliable difference between integrated treatment and the control conditions on SUD outcomes and only a marginally significant difference favoring integrated treatment for PTSD outcomes.

The reviews by Berenz and Coffey (2012), McCauley et al. (2012), and van Dam et al. (2012) were all narrative and divided the interventions into those that did and those that did not involve specific trauma exposure elements. Each of the reviews concluded that the non–trauma-focused CBT interventions did not confer added benefit compared with standard SUD interventions either with regard to substance use outcomes or PTSD. Only a handful of studies involving trauma-focused interventions have been published to date, and the consensus across the reviews is that patients who completed the protocols reported reduced PTSD, although generally not reduced SUD behaviors relative to control conditions. The exposure-based interventions were, however, also typically associated with high dropout.

A recent randomized clinical trial that was not included in the reviews compared Concurrent Treatment of PTSD and Substance Use Disorders Using Prolonged Exposure (COPE) plus SUD treatment to SUD treatment alone and also found high dropout rates such that just over half actually received any exposure sessions and only 18.2% completed all 13 sessions (Mills et al., 2012). There was a significant Group × Time interaction in the intent-to-treat analyses, with those randomized to COPE reporting less severe PTSD relative to the standard SUD treatment comparison group at the 9-month follow-up. There was not, however, a significant effect of treatment assignment on substance use outcomes, although both groups reduced the number of drug classes used, and the rate of substance dependence fell significantly from baseline to 9-month follow-up. Two other randomized clinical trials are currently evaluating integrated trauma-focused exposure-based interventions for PTSD–SUD (Coffey, Schumacher, & Stasiewicz, 2012; Riggs & Foa, 2008).

All four reviews noted that methodological limitations, including uncontrolled trials, small sample sizes, and unblinded assessment, hamper our ability to determine whether integrated treatments for PTSD–SUD hold promise for better outcomes than nonintegrated treatments. It is noteworthy that SUD treatment alone appears to be beneficial for both SUD and PTSD outcomes, and Torchalla et al. (2012) suggested that despite the strong theoretical rationale for integrated treatments, it is possible that SUD treatments help to alleviate PTSD through a variety of nonspecific factors (e.g., therapeutic alliance) or perhaps generalization of SUD-oriented skills to trauma-related issues. There is also early indication that treatment focused only on PTSD could be beneficial for people with PTSD–AUD (Kaysen et al., 2014). Preliminary evidence comes from a large open-trial evaluation of an empirically supported treatment for PTSD, cognitive processing therapy (CPT; Resick, Nishith, Weaver, Astin, & Feurer, 2002), in a Veterans Affairs clinical setting that compared veterans with PTSD with no history of AUD, past AUD, and current AUD. The three groups were not found to differ with regard to the number of sessions attended (average was nine), and all three groups reported significant decreases in PTSD and depression severity. Substance use was not reported. Kaysen and Simpson have a randomized clinical trial underway comparing CPT, relapse prevention, and an assessment-only waitlist condition for individuals with current PTSD and an AUD. The trial involves daily symptom monitoring during the treatment phase to evaluate the sequence of symptom changes associated with the two active conditions relative to the control condition (National Institutes of Health/National Institute on Alcohol Abuse and Alcoholism, grant no. R01AA020252-01).

In summary, the empirical literature regarding how best to intervene psychotherapeutically for individuals with co-occurring PTSD–SUD is in its infancy. Rigorous, well-designed clinical trials are necessary to determine whether some form of integrated treatment can succeed in reducing both PTSD and SUD behaviors or whether treatments focused on SUD or on PTSD are sufficient. In the meantime, it is noteworthy that standard SUD treatments appear to be as beneficial for reducing both substance use and PTSD symptoms as tailored integrated treatments that are not exposure-based, which offers some measure of assurance that interventions that are already widely available do have some utility in addressing this commonly seen comorbidity.

INTEGRATING PSYCHOTHERAPY AND PHARMACOTHERAPY

The issue of how to combine integrated behavioral interventions plus SUD-specific medications for co-occurring PTSD and SUD also demands further investigation. A randomized controlled trial of an eight-session manualized smoking cessation intervention for individuals with co-occurring PTSD and tobacco use disorder, which strongly encouraged the use of smoking cessation medications, demonstrated that prolonged abstinence rates from tobacco could be effectively doubled by integrating the treatments so that both are delivered by a single provider, versus sending PTSD patients to a smoking cessation clinic (McFall et al., 2010). The patients receiving integrated care had reductions in PTSD symptoms equivalent to reductions achieved by patients with the interventions separated. Patients in integrated care received significantly more days of smoking cessation medications, which mediated nearly 10% of the observed treatment effect. This model of success at integration of PTSD and SUD treatment, along with SUD pharmacotherapy, encourages investigation of its application to other co-occurring SUDs.

A recently completed clinical trial enrolled participants with co-occurring PTSD and alcohol dependence and randomized them to one of four study conditions: (a) prolonged exposure therapy plus naltrexone 100 mg/day; (b) prolonged exposure therapy plus placebo; (c) supportive counseling plus naltrexone 100 mg/day; (d) supportive counseling plus placebo (Foa et al., 2013). All participants showed large decreases in number of days using alcohol, with naltrexone-treated participants using on significantly fewer days than placebo-treated participants. All participants also showed large decreases in PTSD symptoms without any noted differences between conditions. This study also supports the idea that treatments for PTSD and SUD can be successfully delivered in an integrated fashion.

SIMULTANEOUS PHARMACOTHERAPY FOR SUD AND PTSD

In addition to integrating psychotherapies, the notion of using a single medication or combination of medications for pharmacologic management of both disorders simultaneously holds some intrigue. The potential promise of topiramate has already been mentioned. The antihypertensive medication prazosin, which blocks alpha-1 adrenergic receptors, has been studied for more than a decade as a treatment for PTSD-related nightmares and other symptoms (Raskind et al., 2007) and has come into fairly widespread use. In a small, double-blind, placebo-controlled trial, prazosin significantly reduced alcohol use in men with alcohol dependence but without PTSD, suggesting that it may have independent efficacy for alcohol dependence (Simpson et al., 2009). Trials are now underway to explore the efficacy of prazosin for patients with co-occurring alcohol dependence and PTSD. Sertraline is an FDA-approved pharmacotherapy for PTSD. Sertraline and naltrexone combined have efficacy for co-occurring depression and AUD (Pettinati et al., 2010), raising the question of what this combination might do for co-occurring PTSD and AUD.

CONCLUSIONS AND CLINICAL MANAGEMENT

In conclusion, some promising avenues are being explored to find the most effective and most parsimonious ways to combine and integrate pharmacotherapies and psychotherapies for co-occurring PTSD and SUD, but definitive answers await additional investigation. At this juncture, a patient with co-occurring PTSD and SUD should receive appropriate pharmacotherapy for the specific SUD being addressed and appropriate pharmacotherapy for PTSD. Additionally, the patient should receive an evidence-based psychotherapy for at least one of the conditions initially, perhaps determined by patient and provider preference, and then receive psychotherapy for the other disorder if signs and symptoms of the other disorder remain poorly controlled.

REFERENCES

American Psychiatric Association. (2013). *Diagnostic and statistical manual of mental disorders* (5th ed.). Arlington, VA: Author.

Berenz, E. C., & Coffey, S. F. (2012). Treatment of co-occurring posttraumatic stress disorder and substance use disorders. *Current Psychiatry Reports, 14,* 469–477. doi:10.1007/s11920-012-0300-0

Blanco, C., Xu, Y., Brady, K., Pérez-Fuentes, G., Okuda, M., & Wang, S. (2013). Comorbidity of posttraumatic stress disorder with alcohol dependence among US adults: Results from National Epidemiological Survey on Alcohol and Related Conditions. *Drug and Alcohol Dependence, 132,* 630–608.

Bradley, K. A., DeBenedetti, A. F., Volk, R. J., Williams, E. C., Frank, D., & Kivlahan, D. R. (2007). AUDIT–C as a brief screen for alcohol misuse in primary care. *Alcoholism: Clinical and Experimental Research, 31,* 1208–1217. doi:10.1111/j.1530-0277.2007.00403.x

Campbell, A. R., & Anderson, K. D. (2010). Mental health stability in veterans with posttraumatic stress disorder receiving varenicline. *American Journal of Health-System Pharmacy, 67,* 1832–1837. doi:10.2146/ajhp100196

Centers for Disease Control and Prevention. (2014). *Drug overdose in the United States: Fact sheet.* Retrieved from http://www.cdc.gov/homeandrecreationalsafety/overdose/facts.html

Coffey, S. F., Schumacher, J. A., & Stasiewicz, P. R. (2012, June). *Prolonged exposure for the treatment of PTSD in a PTSD-alcohol dependent sample.* Presented at the 35th Annual Scientific Meeting of the Research Society on Alcoholism, San Francisco, CA.

Donovan, B., Padin-Rivera, E., & Kowaliw, S. (2001). "Transcend": Initial outcomes from a posttraumatic stress disorder/substance abuse treatment program. *Journal of Traumatic Stress, 14,* 757–772. doi:10.1023/A:1013094206154

Donovan, D. M., Kivlahan, D. R., Doyle, S. R., Longabaugh, R., & Greenfield, S. F. (2006). Concurrent validity of the Alcohol Use Disorders Identification

Test (AUDIT) and AUDIT zones in defining levels of severity among outpatients with alcohol dependence in the COMBINE study. *Addiction, 101,* 1696–1704. doi:10.1111/j.1360-0443.2006.01606.x

Fiore, M. C., Jaén, C. R., & Baker, T. B. (2008). *Clinical Practice Guideline. Treating tobacco use and dependence: 2008 update.* Rockville, MD: U.S. Department of Health and Human Services, Public Health Service.

Foa, E. B., Yusko, D. A., McLean, C. P., Suvak, M. K., Bux, D. A., Jr., Oslin, D., . . . Volpicelli, J. (2013). Concurrent naltrexone and prolonged exposure therapy for patients with comorbid alcohol dependence and PTSD: A randomized clinical trial. *JAMA, 310,* 488–495. doi:10.1001/jama.2013.8268

Garza, D., Murphy, M., Tseng, L. J., Riordan, H. J., & Chatterjee, A. (2011). A double-blind randomized placebo-controlled pilot study of neuropsychiatric adverse events in abstinent smokers treated with varenicline or placebo. *Biological Psychiatry, 69,* 1075–1082. doi:10.1016/j.biopsych.2010.12.005

Gonzales, K., Roeber, J., Kanny, D., Tran, A., Saiki, C., Johnson, H., . . . Geiger, S. D. (2014). Alcohol-attributable deaths and years of potential life lost—11 states, 2006–2010. *MMWR Morbidity and Mortality Weekly Report, 63,* 213–216.

Green, A. I., Drake, R. E., Brunette, M. F., & Noordsy, D. L. (2007). Schizophrenia and co-occurring substance use disorder. *The American Journal of Psychiatry, 164,* 402–408. doi:10.1176/appi.ajp.164.3.402

Gunne, L. M., & Gronbladh, L. (1981). The Swedish methadone maintenance program: A controlled study. *Drug and Alcohol Dependence, 7,* 249–256. doi:10.1016/0376-8716(81)90096-X

Hertzberg, M. A., Moore, S. D., Feldman, M. E., & Beckham, J. C. (2001). A preliminary study of bupropion sustained-release for smoking cessation in patients with chronic posttraumatic stress disorder. *Journal of Clinical Psychopharmacology, 21,* 94–98. doi:10.1097/00004714-200102000-00017

Himelhoch, S., Weber, E., Medoff, D., Charlotte, M., Clayton, S., Wilson, C., . . . Benford, J. (2012). Posttraumatic stress disorder and one-year outcome in methadone maintenance treatment. *The American Journal on Addictions, 21,* 524–530. doi:10.1111/j.1521-0391.2012.00271.x

Jha, P., Ramasundarahettige, C., Landsman, V., Rostron, B., Thun, M., Anderson, R. N., . . . Peto, R. (2013). 21st-century hazards of smoking and benefits of cessation in the United States. *The New England Journal of Medicine, 368,* 341–350. doi:10.1056/NEJMsa1211128

Kakko, J., Svanborg, K. D., Kreek, M. J., & Heilig, M. (2003). 1-year retention and social function after buprenorphine-assisted relapse prevention treatment for heroin dependence in Sweden: A randomised, placebo-controlled trial. *The Lancet, 361,* 662–668. doi:10.1016/S0140-6736(03)12600-1

Kaysen, D., Schumm, J., Pedersen, E. R., Seim, R. W., Bedard-Gilligan, M., & Chard, K. (2014). Cognitive processing therapy for veterans with comorbid PTSD and Alcohol Use Disorders. *Addictive Behaviors, 39*, 420–427.

Kessler, R. C., Sonnega, A., Bromet, E., Hughes, M., & Nelson, C. B. (1995). Posttraumatic stress disorder in the National Comorbidity Survey. *Archives of General Psychiatry, 52*, 1048–1060. doi:10.1001/archpsyc.1995.03950240066012

Krupitsky, E., Nunes, E. V., Ling, W., Illeperuma, A., Gastfriend, D. R., & Silverman, B. L. (2011). Injectable extended-release naltrexone for opioid dependence: A double-blind, placebo-controlled, multicentre randomised trial. *The Lancet, 377*, 1506–1513. doi:10.1016/S0140-6736(11)60358-9

McCauley, J. L., Killeen, T., Gros, D. F., Brady, K. T., & Back, S. E. (2012). Posttraumatic stress disorder and co-occurring substance use disorders: Advances in assessment and treatment. *Clinical Psychology: Science and Practice, 19*, 283–304. doi:10.1111/cpsp.12006

McFall, M., Saxon, A. J., Malte, C. A., Chow, B., Bailey, S., Baker, D. G., . . . Lavori, P. W. (2010). Integrating tobacco cessation into mental health care for post-traumatic stress disorder: A randomized controlled trial. *JAMA, 304*, 2485–2493. doi:10.1001/jama.2010.1769

Mills, K. L., Teesson, M., Back, S. E., Brady, K. T., Baker, A. L., Hopwood, S., . . . Ewer, P. L. (2012). Integrated exposure-based therapy for co-occurring posttraumatic stress disorder and substance dependence. *JAMA, 308*, 690–699. doi:10.1001/jama.2012.9071

Mitchell, J. M., O'Neil, J. P., Janabi, M., Marks, S. M., Jagust, W. J., & Fields, H. L. (2012). Alcohol consumption induces endogenous opioid release in the human orbitofrontal cortex and nucleus accumbens. *Science Translational Medicine, 4*, 116ra6.

Najavits, L. M., Harned, M. S., Gallop, J., Butler, S. F., Barber, J. P., & Thase, M. E. (2007). Six-month treatment outcomes of cocaine-dependent patients with and without PTSD in a multisite national trial. *Journal of Studies on Alcohol and Drugs, 68*, 353–361.

Norman, S. B., Myers, U. S., Wilkins, K. C., Goldsmith, A. A., Hristova, V., Huang, Z., . . . Robinson, S. K. (2012). Review of biological mechanisms and pharmacological treatments of comorbid PTSD and substance use disorder. *Neuropharmacology, 62*, 542–551. doi:10.1016/j.neuropharm.2011.04.032

Petrakis, I. L., Poling, J., Levinson, C., Nich, C., Carroll, K., Ralevski, E., & Rounsaville, B. (2006). Naltrexone and disulfiram in patients with alcohol dependence and comorbid post-traumatic stress disorder. *Biological Psychiatry, 60*, 777–783. doi:10.1016/j.biopsych.2006.03.074

Pettinati, H. M., Oslin, D. W., Kampman, K. M., Dundon, W. D., Xie, H., Gallis, T. L., . . . O'Brien, C. P. (2010). A double-blind, placebo-controlled trial combining sertraline and naltrexone for treating co-occurring depression and alcohol dependence. *The American Journal of Psychiatry, 167,* 668–675. doi:10.1176/appi.ajp.2009.08060852

Raskind, M. A., Peskind, E. R., Hoff, D. J., Hart, K. L., Holmes, H. A., Warren, D., . . . McFall, M. E. (2007). A parallel group placebo controlled study of prazosin for trauma nightmares and sleep disturbance in combat veterans with post-traumatic stress disorder. *Biological Psychiatry, 61,* 928–934. doi:10.1016/j.biopsych.2006.06.032

Resick, P. A., Nishith, P., Weaver, T. L., Astin, M. C., & Feurer, C. A. (2002). A comparison of cognitive processing therapy with prolonged exposure and a waiting condition for the treatment of chronic posttraumatic stress disorder in female rape victims. *Journal of Consulting and Clinical Psychology, 70,* 867–879. doi:10.1037/0022-006X.70.4.867

Riggs, D. S., & Foa, E. B. (2008). Treatment for co-morbid posttraumatic stress disorder and substance use disorders. In S. H. Stewart & P. J. Conrad (Eds.), *Anxiety and substance use disorders: The vicious cycle of comorbidity* (pp. 119–137). New York, NY: Springer. doi:10.1007/978-0-387-74290-8_7

Saladin, M. E., Brady, K. T., Dansky, B. S., & Kilpatrick, D. G. (1995). Understanding comorbidity between PTSD and substance use disorder: Two preliminary investigations. *Addictive Behaviors, 20,* 643–655. doi:10.1016/0306-4603(95)00024-7

Schneider, B. (2009). Substance use disorders and risk for completed suicide. *Archives of Suicide Research, 13,* 303–316. doi:10.1080/13811110903263191

Simpson, T. L., Saxon, A. J., Meredith, C. W., Malte, C. A., McBride, B., Ferguson, L. C., . . . Raskind, M. (2009). A pilot trial of the alpha-1 adrenergic antagonist, prazosin, for alcohol dependence. *Alcoholism: Clinical and Experimental Research, 33,* 255–263. doi:10.1111/j.1530-0277.2008.00807.x

Smith, P. C., Schmidt, S. M., Allensworth-Davies, D., & Saitz, R. (2010). A single-question screening test for drug use in primary care. *Archives of Internal Medicine, 170,* 1155–1160. doi:10.1001/archinternmed.2010.140

Torchalla, I., Nosen, L., Rostam, H., & Allen, P. (2012). Integrated treatment programs for individuals with concurrent substance use disorders and trauma experiences: A systematic review and meta-analysis. *Journal of Substance Abuse Treatment, 42,* 65–77. doi:10.1016/j.jsat.2011.09.001

Triffleman, E., Carroll, K., & Kellogg, S. (1999). Substance dependence posttraumatic stress disorder therapy: An integrated cognitive-behavioral approach. *Journal of Substance Abuse Treatment, 17,* 3–14. doi:10.1016/S0740-5472(98)00067-1 van Dam, D., Vedel, E., Ehring, T., & Emmelkamp, P. M. (2012). Psychological treatments for concurrent posttraumatic stress disorder and substance use disorder: A systematic review. *Clinical Psychology Review, 32*, 202–214. doi:10.1016/j.cpr.2012.01.004

Yeh, M. S., Mari, J. J., Costa, M. C., Andreoli, S. B., Bressan, R. A., & Mello, M. F. (2011). A double-blind randomized controlled trial to study the efficacy of topiramate in a civilian sample of PTSD. *CNS Neuroscience & Therapeutics, 17*, 305–310. doi:10.1111/j.1755-5949.2010.00188.x

10

Treating PTSD in Older Adults

Joan M. Cook, Ahsan Naseem, and Steven R. Thorp

The goals of this chapter are to note the prevalence of posttraumatic stress disorder (PTSD) in older adults, provide information on the longitudinal course of PTSD, discuss differences between younger and older trauma survivors, and provide information on effective pharmacotherapy and psychotherapy for PTSD in the older population. This information is important for numerous reasons, including the increase in the number and proportion of older adults in the United States. Compared with what is known about trauma and PTSD in other age groups, relatively little is known about this disorder in older individuals. A review of nearly 10,000 PTSD articles published since 1980 found that 82% of articles were focused on a general adult population, more than 16% were

This chapter was coauthored by an employee of the United States government as part of official duty and is considered to be in the public domain. Any views expressed herein do not necessarily represent the views of the United States government, and the author's participation in the work is not meant to serve as an official endorsement.

http://dx.doi.org/10.1037/14522-011
A Practical Guide to PTSD Treatment: Pharmacological and Psychotherapeutic Approaches,
N. C. Bernardy and M. J. Friedman (Editors)
Copyright © 2015 by the American Psychological Association. All rights reserved.

focused on children, and less than 2% were focused on older adults (Priest et al., 2010). Although it is thought that PTSD is not substantially different in older adults, some symptoms do appear less intense. Some symptoms of PTSD, however, may be underdetected in older adults. Thus, it is likely that PTSD is underrecognized and undertreated in this population and that lack of recognition or misattribution of symptoms can have a serious impact on the provision of effective care.

DIFFERENCES IN OLDER PTSD PATIENTS

The biggest difference is that lifetime rates of PTSD appear to be lower for older adults than younger adults by about half—somewhere in the 3.5% range in older versus approximately 6.8% in the general population. The epidemiological studies that do include older adults have shown that lifetime PTSD prevalence is lower in older as opposed to younger or middle-aged adults. Lifetime rates in older adults have been similar across samples, including rates of 2.5% (Kessler et al., 2005), 2.7% (de Vries & Olff, 2009), 3.1% (Spitzer et al., 2008), and 4.5% (Pietrzak et al., 2012b). This compares with lifetime rates of PTSD of 6.8% in the general adult population (Kessler et al., 2005). Twelve-month PTSD prevalence in this population ranges from 0.2% (Creamer & Parslow, 2008) to 1.5% (Spitzer et al., 2008).

Although not a widely investigated phenomenon in older adults, partial PTSD criteria are also met in a substantial proportion of older adults (5.5% in Pietrzak et al., 2012b, and 13.1% in van Zelst, de Beurs, Beekman, Deeg, & van Dyck, 2003). In community-residing older veterans, less than 1% met full PTSD criteria, and nearly 10% had partial PTSD (Schnurr, Spiro, Vielhauer, Findler, & Hamblen, 2002). Estimates of PTSD derived from clinical samples, such as those in psychiatric or medical settings, are understandably higher, ranging from 8% in those who never sought psychiatric treatment to 80% in those who had previously sought psychiatric services (e.g., Blake et al., 1990).

In samples of older veterans, there is a strong association between PTSD symptoms and self-reported physical health, which is not mediated by smoking or alcohol use (Schnurr & Spiro, 1999). Older adults with PTSD were more likely than older adults who were trauma-exposed without PTSD to report worse physical functioning and to report being diagnosed with hypertension, angina pectoris, tachycardia, other heart disease, stomach ulcers, gastritis, and arthritis (Pietrzak, Goldstein, Southwick, & Grant, 2012a). There is also a strong association between PTSD and physician-diagnosed disorders, such as arterial, lower gastrointestinal, and musculoskeletal disorders (Schnurr, Spiro, & Paris, 2000).

The lower rates of PTSD and other trauma-related distress in older as opposed to younger or middle-aged adults may be due to a number of factors. For example, younger adults may recognize or acknowledge more symptoms because of less perceived stigma regarding mental health. Additionally, older adults may be more likely to label any difficulties as somatic complaints and thus seek medical as opposed to mental health care. Furthermore, age at the time of trauma may be a factor influencing reporting or experiencing symptoms in that older adults who were traumatized earlier in life may have been socialized not to discuss mental health problems outside of the home. Last, less distress in older adults may be due to normal aging processes, maturity in coping strategies, and the passage of time lessening symptom severity.

Experiences seen as potentially traumatic and identified by older adults are relatively consistent. Unexpected death or serious illness or injury to someone close to them and their own serious illnesses are often identified as the worst stressful events (Breslau et al., 1998; Breslau, Peterson, Poisson, Schultz, & Lucia, 2004; Spitzer et al., 2008).

LONGITUDINAL COURSE OF PTSD

Relatively little is known about the course of PTSD over the lifetime. One retrospective report from a snowball sample of former prisoners of war (POWs) found that for most individuals (60%), symptoms are perceived to wax and wane across the life span (Zeiss & Dickman, 1989). The rest report being either relatively symptom free (20%) or continuously troubled (20%). Another investigation primarily obtained retrospective data on the course of PTSD but also included a 4-year longitudinal data piece when older former POWs were in old age. The majority of men reported an immediate onset and gradual decline of PTSD symptoms after the war, followed by a return of higher PTSD symptom levels in later life (Port, Engdahl, & Frazier, 2001). The apparent ebb and flow of symptoms across the life course and the noted increase or recognition in old age may be due to developmental life changes. Older adults are typically at increased risk for physical health problems and functional status loss. Many also experience losses in occupational, social, and familial roles as a consequence of disability, retirement, and bereavement. Some individuals may experience delayed onset of PTSD until older adulthood, although for the majority, it can be more accurately labeled as delayed recognition (Hiskey, Luckie, Davies, & Brewin, 2008).

The relationships among traumatic exposure, PTSD, and cognitive functioning in late life are poorly understood. Several case reports indicate that dementia may exacerbate existing PTSD symptoms (e.g., Johnston, 2000). In addition, of 181,000 older veterans followed over a 6-year period, those with PTSD were more than twice as likely to develop dementia (Yaffe et al., 2010). However, PTSD and dementia may share a third variable, intelligence, which may account for these correlations (Pitman, 2010).

PHARMACOLOGICAL TREATMENTS

The empirical literature offers comparatively little guidance in regard to pharmacotherapy for PTSD in older as opposed to younger adults. Most of the pharmacotherapy studies for PTSD have not included older adults, and often when older adults were included, age comparisons were not conducted. Two studies have been conducted expressly with older adults (Hamner, Deitsch, Brodrick, Ulmer, & Lorberbaum, 2003; Peskind, Bonner, Hoff, & Raskind, 2003). Both prazosin (Peskind et al., 2003) and the atypical antipsychotic quetiapine (Hamner et al., 2003) were found to reduce PTSD symptoms in older individuals.

Some experts believe that tricyclic antidepressants may work better than selective serotonin reuptake inhibitors for more chronic PTSD, such as that often seen in older veterans (Friedman, Davidson, Mellman, & Southwick, 2000). However the potential side effect profile of this class of medications may not be optimal for older adults with medical issues such as hypertension or cardiac disease.

Although benzodiazepines have been found to decrease hyperarousal symptoms (e.g., insomnia, anxiety, irritability), they do not lead to significant reductions in reexperiencing or avoidance symptoms. Despite well-known adverse effects (e.g., cognitive impairment, increased risk of falls) and the availability of safer, effective medications, many providers continue to prescribe benzodiazepines to older adults. This has been identified as a public health problem (Cook, Marshall, Masci, & Coyne, 2007). Although well intentioned, many physicians tend to minimize the risks of benzodiazepines in older individuals and also remain skeptical about the possibilities for successful taper or discontinuation in older patients with long-term use and previous failed attempts. Strategies to address this potential dilemma include increasing practitioner skill level in facilitating discontinuation and preventing new cases of potential benzodiazepine dependency through improved patient education and vigilant monitoring of prescription renewal.

A number of age-related concerns should be taken into account when choosing psychotropic medications for PTSD in older adults. With aging comes changes in anatomy and physiology that may complicate efficacy of medications. For example, absorption rates and distribution are altered (e.g., reduction in lean muscle mass, increase in total body fat). Many older adults take numerous medications concurrently, and polypharmacy issues need to be taken into account in the administration and dosing of PTSD pharmacotherapies. Antipsychotics (typical and atypical), mood stabilizers, and alpha-antagonists should be used cautiously with older adults with PTSD because there are risks for toxicity and possibly increased rates of mortality (Jacobson, Pies, & Katz, 2007).

PSYCHOTHERAPY TREATMENTS

The psychotherapy literature primarily comprises single or multiple case studies or group therapy descriptions in the treatment of distal trauma-related issues (i.e., Holocaust and combat; for a review, see Cook & O'Donnell, 2005). There may be special considerations about psychotherapy with older adults due to cardiovascular functioning or cognitive issues.

The literature indicates that relaxation training and cognitive behavioral techniques (including exposure) have been successful and well tolerated for most non-PTSD anxiety disorders in older adults (for a review, see Thorp, Ayers, Nuevo, Stoddard, Sorrell, & Wetherell, 2009). Two studies investigated the role of age on clinical outcomes among individuals with PTSD. In one randomized controlled trial of 145 sexual assault survivors with PTSD, older women in prolonged exposure (PE; Foa, Hembree, & Rothbaum, 2007) and younger women in cognitive processing therapy (CPT; Resick & Schnicke, 1993) had the best outcomes (Rizvi, Vogt, & Resick, 2009). The authors suggested that this may be due to challenges in changing chronic maladaptive cognitions in older individuals, but this was a fairly young sample, and more psychotherapy outcome research with an older population is needed. In the other study (Chard, Schumm, Owens, & Cottingham, 2010), 51 veterans who returned from the current wars in Iraq and Afghanistan (mean age 31 years) were compared with 50 Vietnam veterans (mean age 59) after treatment with CPT. The younger cohort attended fewer sessions of treatment. After controlling for number of sessions attended and pretreatment clinician-rated PTSD severity scores, the younger cohort had lower posttreatment PTSD severity scores. This suggests that older age or a longer duration of PTSD symptoms may limit treatment response.

The psychotherapies with the strongest support for treating PTSD in the general population are exposure therapies (Bradley, Greene, Russ, Dutra, & Westen, 2005). Although the use of intensive trauma processing methods such as exposure in the older population has been questioned because they may lead to increased autonomic arousal and decreased cognitive performance (e.g., Hyer, & Woods, 1998), the tolerance and effect of increased physiological arousal that can accompany trauma processing remains an open empirical question. In the absence of empirical data, it seems reasonable to proceed with appropriate caution and monitor those older adults who are at great risk from high arousal, such as those with serious cardiac or respiratory problems.

Findings from two pilot studies on the use of exposure therapies for older veterans with PTSD have been reported. In one study (Gamito et al., 2010), 10 older combat veterans were randomly assigned to virtual reality exposure therapy ($n = 5$), "exposure in imagination" (which was not operationalized; $n = 2$), or wait list ($n = 3$). There were improvements in clinician-rated PTSD severity following the virtual reality exposure (8% reduction) and the exposure in imagination (1% reduction), compared with a 6% reduction for veterans on the wait list. In another study (Thorp, Stein, Jeste, Patterson, & Wetherell, 2012), eleven older male veterans with primarily combat-related PTSD were enrolled in an open trial of 12 sessions of PE. The results were promising in regard to tolerance and symptom reduction (a 49% reduction in clinician-rated PTSD severity following PE, compared with a 13% reduction for those receiving treatment as usual). A randomized controlled trial is underway (Steven R. Thorp, principal investigator) comparing the efficacy of 12 sessions of relaxation training with that of PE for older male veterans. The application of empirically based treatments for PTSD, such as PE and CPT, warrants additional investigation in older adults.

The role that cognitive impairment may play in the provision of psychotherapy in older veterans is unknown. Cognitive impairment may lower the threshold for emotional response to cues or "triggers" for PTSD symptoms and disinhibit subsequent problem behaviors. In addition, because most psychotherapies are learning-based interventions, older veterans with cognitive impairment may not respond as well to treatment. Among veterans with PTSD, those with poor verbal memory and narrative encoding deficits were more likely to be nonresponsive to eight sessions of cognitive behavioral therapy than those without PTSD

(Wild & Gur, 2008). These differences were not due to intelligence, attention, PTSD severity, depression, time since trauma, or substance misuse. Clinical management of PTSD in those with cognitive impairments may require adding environmental or caregiver interventions to standard psychotherapy protocols.

CONCLUSION

A number of clinical implications and training recommendations exist for working with older PTSD adults. Health care professionals should receive ongoing and routine education and training about the apparent association among past trauma, PTSD, cognitive impairment, and behavioral problems in older adults (Cook, Ruzek, & Cassidy, 2003). Ideally, clinicians should be able to accurately assess and treat these potential problems (and realize when referrals to specialists are indicated). There is some evidence to suggest that psychotherapy and pharmacotherapy can be helpful for older adults with PTSD, but continued research in epidemiology, course, treatment, and cognitive limitations will prove invaluable for older adults in the years to come.

REFERENCES

Blake, D. B., Keane, T. M., Wine, P. R., Mora, C., Taylor, K. L., & Lyons, J. A. (1990). Prevalence of PTSD symptoms in combat veterans seeking medical treatment. *Journal of Traumatic Stress, 3*, 15–27. doi:10.1002/jts.2490030103

Bradley, R., Greene, J., Russ, E., Dutra, L., & Westen, D. (2005). A multidimensional meta-analysis of psychotherapy for PTSD. *The American Journal of Psychiatry, 162*, 214–227.

Breslau, N., Kessler, R., Chilcoat, H., Schultz, L., Davis, G., & Andreski, P. (1998). Trauma and posttraumatic stress disorder in the community: The 1996 Detroit Area Survey of Trauma. *Archives of General Psychiatry, 55*, 626–632. doi:10.1001/archpsyc.55.7.626

Breslau, N., Peterson, E. L., Poisson, L. M., Schultz, L. R., & Lucia, V. C. (2004). Estimating post-traumatic stress disorder in the community: Lifetime perspective and the impact of typical traumatic events. *Psychological Medicine, 34*, 889–898. doi:10.1017/S0033291703001612

Chard, K. M., Schumm, J. A., Owens, G. P., & Cottingham, S. M. (2010). A comparison of OEF and OIF veterans and Vietnam veterans receiving cognitive processing therapy. *Journal of Traumatic Stress, 23*, 25–32.

Cook, J. M., Marshall, R., Masci, C., & Coyne, J. C. (2007). Physicians' perspectives on prescribing benzodiazepines for older adults: A qualitative study. *Journal of General Internal Medicine, 22*, 303–307. doi:10.1007/s11606-006-0021-3

Cook, J. M., & O'Donnell, C. (2005). Assessment and psychological treatment of posttraumatic stress disorder in older adults. *Journal of Geriatric Psychiatry and Neurology, 18*, 61–71. doi:10.1177/0891988705276052

Cook, J. M., Ruzek, J. I., & Cassidy, E. L. (2003). Post-traumatic stress disorder and cognitive impairment in older adults: Awareness and recognition of a possible association. *Psychiatric Services, 54*, 1223–1225. doi:10.1176/appi.ps.54.9.1223

Creamer, M., & Parslow, R. (2008). Trauma exposure and posttraumatic stress disorder in the elderly: A community prevalence study. *The American Journal of Geriatric Psychiatry, 16*, 853–856. doi:10.1097/01.JGP.0000310785.36837.85

de Vries, G. J., & Olff, M. (2009). The lifetime prevalence of traumatic events and posttraumatic stress disorder in the Netherlands. *Journal of Traumatic Stress, 22*, 259–267. doi:10.1002/jts.20429

Foa, E. B., Hembree, E. A., & Rothbaum, B. O. (2007). *Prolonged exposure therapy for PTSD: Emotional processing of traumatic experiences—therapist guide.* New York, NY: Oxford University Press.

Friedman, M. J., Davidson, J. R. T., Mellman, T. A., & Southwick, S. M. (2000). Pharmacotherapy. In E. Foa, T. M. Keane, & M. J. Friedman (Eds.), *Effective treatments for PTSD: Practice guidelines from the International Society for Traumatic Stress Studies* (pp. 326–329). New York, NY: Guilford Press.

Gamito, P., Oliveira, J., Rosa, P., Morais, D., Duarte, N., Oliveira, S., & Saraiva, T. (2010). PTSD elderly war veterans: A clinical controlled pilot study. *Cyberpsychology, Behavior, and Social Networking, 13*, 43–48. doi:10.1089/cyber.2009.0237

Hamner, M. B., Deitsch, S. E., Brodrick, P. S., Ulmer, H. G., & Lorberbaum, J. P. (2003). Quetiapine treatment in patients with posttraumatic stress disorder: An open trial of adjunctive therapy. *Journal of Clinical Psychopharmacology, 23*, 15–20. doi:10.1097/00004714-200302000-00003

Hiskey, S., Luckie, M., Davies, S., & Brewin, C. R. (2008). The emergence of posttraumatic distress later in life: A review. *Journal of Geriatric Psychiatry and Neurology, 21*, 232–241.

Hyer, L. A., & Woods, M. G. (1998). Phenomenology and treatment of trauma in later life. In V. M. Follette, J. I. Ruzek, & F. R. Abueg (Eds.), *Cognitive-behavioral therapies for trauma* (pp. 383–414). New York, NY: Guilford Press.

Jacobson, S. A., Pies, R. W., & Katz, I. R. (2007). *Clinical manual of geriatric psychopharmacology.* Washington, DC: American Psychiatric Publishing.

Johnston, D. (2000). A series of cases of dementia presenting with PTSD symptoms in World War II combat veterans. *Journal of the American Geriatrics Society, 48,* 70–72.

Kessler, R. C., Berglund, P., Demler, O., Jin, R., Merikangas, K. R., & Walters, E. E. (2005). Lifetime prevalence and age-of-onset distributions of *DSM–IV* disorders in the National Comorbidity Survey Replication [corrected in *Archives of General Psychiatry, 62,* 768]. *Archives of General Psychiatry, 62,* 593–602. doi:10.1001/archpsyc.62.6.593

Peskind, E. R., Bonner, L. T., Hoff, D. J., & Raskind, M. A. (2003). Prazosin reduces trauma-related nightmares in older men with chronic posttraumatic stress disorder. *Journal of Geriatric Psychiatry and Neurology, 16,* 165–171. doi:10.1177/0891988703256050

Pietrzak, R. H., Goldstein, R. B., Southwick, S. M., & Grant, B. F. (2012a). Physical health conditions associated with posttraumatic stress disorder in U.S. older adults: Results from wave 2 of the National Epidemiologic Survey on Alcohol and Related Conditions. *Journal of the American Geriatrics Society, 60,* 296–303. doi:10.1111/j.1532-5415.2011.03788.x

Pietrzak, R. H., Goldstein, R. B., Southwick, S. M., & Grant, B. F. (2012b). Psychiatric comorbidity of full and partial posttraumatic stress disorder among older adults in the United States: Results from wave 2 of the National Epidemiologic Survey on Alcohol and Related Conditions. *The American Journal of Geriatric Psychiatry, 20,* 380–390. doi:10.1097/JGP.0b013e31820d92e7

Pitman, R. K. (2010). Posttraumatic stress disorder and dementia: What is the origin of the association? *JAMA, 303,* 2287–2288. doi:10.1001/jama.2010.767

Port, C. L., Engdahl, B., & Frazier, P. (2001). A longitudinal and retrospective study of PTSD among older POWs. *The American Journal of Psychiatry, 158,* 1474–1479. doi:10.1176/appi.ajp.158.9.1474

Priest, E. G., Dahlin, K. M., Lucas, C. M., Stevens, J. M., Rivas, T. E., Lightman, N. S., ... Dalenberg, C. J. (2010, August). *Biologically oriented publications in child and adult PTSD research: Emerging trends.* Paper presented at the 118th Annual American Psychological Association National Convention, San Diego, CA.

Resick, P. A., & Schnicke, M. K. (1993). *Cognitive processing therapy for rape victims: A treatment manual.* Newbury Park, CA: Sage.

Rizvi, S. L., Vogt, D. S., & Resick, P. A. (2009). Cognitive and affective predictors of treatment outcome in cognitive processing therapy and prolonged exposure for posttraumatic stress disorder. *Behaviour Research and Therapy, 47,* 737–743. doi:10.1016/j.brat.2009.06.003

Schnurr, P. P., & Spiro, A., III. (1999). Combat exposure, posttraumatic stress disorder symptoms, and health behaviors as predictors of self-reported physical health in older veterans. *Journal of Nervous and Mental Disease, 187,* 353–359. doi:10.1097/00005053-199906000-00004

Schnurr, P. P., Spiro, A., III, & Paris, A. H. (2000). Physician-diagnosed medical disorders in relation to PTSD symptoms in older male military veterans. *Health Psychology, 19,* 91–97. doi:10.1037/0278-6133.19.1.91

Schnurr, P. P., Spiro, A., Vielhauer, M. J., Findler, M. N., & Hamblen, J. L. (2002). Trauma in the lives of older men: Findings from the Normative Aging Study. *Journal of Clinical Geropsychology, 8,* 175–187. doi:10.1023/A:1015992110544

Spitzer, C., Barnow, S., Völzke, H., John, U., Freyberger, H. J., & Grabe, H. J. (2008). Trauma and posttraumatic stress disorder in the elderly: Findings from a German community study. *Journal of Clinical Psychiatry, 69,* 693–700. doi:10.4088/JCP.v69n0501

Thorp, S. R., Ayers, C. R., Nuevo, R., Stoddard, J. A., Sorrell, J. T., & Wetherell, J. L. (2009). Meta-analysis comparing different behavioral treatments for late-life anxiety. *The American Journal of Geriatric Psychiatry, 17,* 105–115. doi:10.1097/JGP.0b013e31818b3f7e

Thorp, S. R., Stein, M. B., Jeste, D. V., Patterson, T. L., & Wetherell, J. L. (2012). Prolonged exposure therapy for older veterans with posttraumatic stress disorder: Pilot study. *The American Journal of Geriatric Psychiatry, 20,* 276–230. doi:10.1097/JGP.0b013e3182435ee9

van Zelst, W. H., de Beurs, E., Beekman, A. T. F., Deeg, D. J. H., & van Dyck, R. (2003). Prevalence and risk factors of posttraumatic stress disorder in older adults. *Psychotherapy and Psychosomatics, 72,* 333–342. doi:10.1159/000073030

Wild, J., & Gur, R. C. (2008). Verbal memory and treatment response in posttraumatic stress disorder. *The British Journal of Psychiatry, 193,* 254–255. doi:10.1192/bjp.bp.107.045922

Yaffe, K., Vittinghoff, E., Lindquist, K., Barnes, D., Covinsky, K. E., Neylan, T., . . . Marmar, C. (2010). Posttraumatic stress disorder and risk of dementia among U.S. veterans. *Archives of General Psychiatry, 67,* 608–613. doi:10.1001/archgenpsychiatry.2010.61

Zeiss, R. A., & Dickman, H. R. (1989). PTSD 40 years later: Incidence and person-situation correlates in former POWs. *Journal of Clinical Psychology, 45,* 80–87. doi:10.1002/1097-4679(198901)45:1<80::AID-JCLP2270450112>3.0.CO;2-V

11

Challenging Presentations in PTSD

Tonya Masino and Sonya Norman

Posttraumatic stress disorder (PTSD) is sometimes part of a challenging presentation of associated problems and comorbid mental illness. In fact, it is not uncommon for someone with PTSD to have multiple (three or more) Axis I comorbidities (Kessler, Sonnega, Bromet, Hughes, & Nelson, 1995). The presence of certain symptoms and subtypes of PTSD, such as aggression and dissociation, also raises unique challenges. Challenging presentations of PTSD are often associated with greater symptom severity and poorer treatment outcomes for all disorders. In this chapter, we highlight some of the symptoms, associated problems, and comorbidities that can complicate the assessment and management

---

This chapter was coauthored by employees of the United States government as part of official duty and is considered to be in the public domain. Any views expressed herein do not necessarily represent the views of the United States government, and the authors' participation in the work is not meant to serve as an official endorsement.

http://dx.doi.org/10.1037/14522-012
A Practical Guide to PTSD Treatment: Pharmacological and Psychotherapeutic Approaches,
N. C. Bernardy and M. J. Friedman (Editors)
Copyright © 2015 by the American Psychological Association. All rights reserved.

of PTSD, including aggression, dissociative and psychotic symptoms, eating-disordered behaviors, and borderline personality disorder (BPD). We then offer recommendations for assessment, treatment, and future research.

BACKGROUND

Multiple pathways have been proposed to explain the high rates of comorbidity of PTSD with other mental health disorders and associated problems, as well as the often challenging patient profiles that result from these comorbidities. Trauma has been shown to be a risk factor for the development of other psychopathology in addition to PTSD. For example, childhood trauma increases the risk of both dissociation and borderline personality disorder. Conversely, having a mental illness such as schizophrenia can increase the likelihood of exposure to situations in which traumatic events might occur. Shared genetic vulnerabilities may place patients at high risk for the development of both PTSD and other disorders. Emotional dysregulation may be a result of or a contributor to traumatic experiences. Patients with difficulty regulating emotions will often display behaviors associated with both avoidance and poor impulse control. For example, a victim of sexual trauma may develop an eating disorder such as anorexia nervosa either as a maladaptive attempt for self-regulation or as a means of avoiding sexual objectification by masking secondary sexual characteristics. Regardless of the order of onset, comorbid problems and disorders can interact with PTSD to raise unique assessment and treatment challenges.

CHALLENGING SYMPTOMS, ASSOCIATED PROBLEMS, AND COMORBIDITIES

The following sections consider five concerns that present unique challenges in the treatment of PTSD: aggression, dissociation, psychosis, BPD, and eating disorders.

Aggression

Definitions and Prevalence

Aggression is a behavior that is intended to harm an object or another person (Bushman & Huesmann, 2010). Aggression can be physical (e.g., hitting, stabbing someone) or nonphysical (yelling, punching walls). *Violence* is a form of physical aggression that has the potential to inflict serious harm on another person (e.g., using a gun or knife, forcing someone to have sex). The majority of individuals with PTSD do not engage in aggression, and violence is particularly rare. However, because some individuals who develop PTSD after trauma exposure demonstrate new-onset aggression, aggressive behavior (specifically "irritable or aggressive behavior") is included as a symptom in the arousal and reactivity criterion for PTSD in the fifth edition of the *Diagnostic and Statistical Manual of Mental Disorders* (DSM–5; American Psychiatric Association, 2013). Definitive prevalence rates of aggression among individuals with PTSD are not known, in part because of limitations across research studies (e.g., inconsistent definitions of aggression, retrospective data collection). In one study, 17% of veterans with PTSD reported physical aggression in the past year (Jakupcak et al., 2007). Another study found that 33% of veterans seeking treatment for PTSD reported nonphysical or physical aggression (or both) toward their intimate partner in the past year (Taft et al., 2009). Studies that have taken risk factors for aggression other than PTSD into consideration have found that the role of PTSD relative to other risk factors is small. Less is known about rates of aggression among nonveterans with PTSD.

Considerations

A growing body of research, mostly with veteran samples, has identified risk factors for aggression. These include younger age, higher combat exposure, witnessing or being a victim of violence in childhood, committing crimes or violent acts as an adolescent, and co-occurring conditions such as PTSD (particularly hyperarousal symptoms), substance abuse, or depression (Elbogen, Wagner, Calhoun, Fuller, & Kinneer, 2010). Studies of nonveteran samples have also identified psychopathy and personality disorders (e.g., antisocial personality disorder) as risk factors for violence. Protective factors that reduce risk of aggression have also been identified. These include a stable living situation; perception of control over one's life; higher resilience; social support; and having basic needs, such as adequate food or housing, met (Elbogen, Johnson, Wagner, Newton, & Beckham, 2012).

Implications

It is important to carefully assess the known risk factors for aggression and violence among individuals with PTSD. Generally, the greater the number of risk factors someone endorses, the higher their risk of aggression. Violence ideation coupled with high irritability and impulsivity is a particularly concerning combination. Evaluation should include asking about access to weapons or other means to perpetrate violence. Static factors (e.g., age, past history of violence) are important to assess because their presence suggests increased risk, whereas modifiable risk factors (e.g., substance use, homelessness) not only suggest increased risk but can also be targets for intervention.

A collaborative treatment approach to reducing risk and bolstering protective factors including psychiatry, psychotherapy, and case management is recommended. Evidence-based treatments (EBTs) for PTSD, including psychotherapy and pharmacotherapy, can reduce PTSD symptoms that elevate risk of aggression, which can in turn reduce overall risk of aggression. There is preliminary evidence that cognitive behavioral anger management may be helpful in reducing some types of aggression (A. D. Marshall et al., 2010). Atypical antipsychotics have been shown to reduce aggression, impulsivity, and explosiveness in PTSD in some studies (Adetunji et al., 2005). Although this effect is rare, psychotropic medication may increase irritability or dysphoria in some individuals, so patients prescribed medications for PTSD, particularly with high risk of aggression, should be closely monitored for any increase in depression, anger, or aggression. If a patient expresses active or imminent intent or plans to harm others, appropriate emergent intervention, such as proper notifications and hospitalization, should be considered.

Dissociation

Definition and Prevalence

Dissociation is most commonly described as a period of disruption and alteration of consciousness, memory, identity, or body awareness or decreased level of awareness of time or of one's self or surroundings. Although mild dissociation is not uncommon even among nonclinical samples (e.g., when someone drives from point A to point B but does not recall the time that elapsed in between), dissociation becomes of clinical concern when it impairs someone's ability to function safely or when it leads to confusion or disorganization. Studies have shown that dissociative symptoms most commonly experienced by individuals with PTSD include derealization (feeling like experiences are not really happening) and depersonalization (feeling outside of oneself or like the self is not real; Hunter, Sierra, & David, 2004). A dissociative subtype of PTSD was added to DSM–5 to encompass symptoms of derealization and depersonalization not related to substance use or other medical conditions. Studies with Vietnam veterans and civilians with PTSD demonstrate that 15% to 30% of individuals with PTSD meet criteria for the dissociative subtype (Lanius, Brand, Vermetten, Frewen, & Spiegel, 2012). A particularly high rate of dissociative reactions are observed in individuals who experienced prolonged or repeated exposure to trauma such as childhood abuse, sexual abuse, or torture (Zlotnick et al., 1994). In samples from the general population, individuals with high dissociation have far higher rates of PTSD than those with low dissociation (Carlson, Dalenberg, & McDade-Montez, 2012).

Considerations

Dissociation can begin during a traumatic event as a way to cope during the trauma and then continue to occur during stressful situations or even at arbitrary times. A genetic susceptibility to dissociation has been suggested. A growing body of research suggests that individuals with PTSD who exhibit dissociation, compared with those who do not, demonstrate a unique form of emotional dysregulation that involves prefrontal mediated limbic inhibition resulting in emotional overmodulation (Lanius et al., 2012).

Implications

Clinicians and patients may hold beliefs that the patient is unsafe or capable of dangerous acts when dissociating. A thorough evaluation before beginning treatment can help the clinician assess whether there is evidence that such beliefs are true. Individuals who dissociate can benefit from EBTs for PTSD, including prolonged exposure (PE) and cognitive processing therapy (CPT), and effective treatment of PTSD can reduce dissociative symptoms (Hagenaars, van Minnen, & Hoogduin, 2010; Resick, Suvak, Johnides, Mitchell, & Iverson, 2012). However, a growing body of research suggests that those with the dissociative subtype of PTSD may respond to treatment differently from those with low or no dissociation. Dissociation may interfere with habituation, a key process in exposure-based treatments, rendering exposure therapies less effective for individuals who dissociate (Lanius et al., 2012). Cloitre and colleagues (2010) showed that PTSD patients with high dissociation showed greater reductions in dissociation and PTSD symptoms in a two-stepped treatment (affective and interpersonal regulation followed by exposure therapy) compared with affective and interpersonal regulation only or exposure only. Resick and colleagues (2012) found that among women who received CPT in a large clinical trial, women with high dissociation responded most efficiently to CPT–C (trauma-focused cognitive therapy without a written trauma account), whereas women with high dissociation responded most efficiently to CPT that included the written trauma account. There are no medications as of yet that specifically target dissociative symptoms. However, medications targeting PTSD may help alleviate anxiety and hyperarousal, which may trigger dissociation. Paroxetine has been shown to reduce dissociation in a randomized trial of patients with PTSD (A. D. Marshall et al., 2010). Benzodiazepines may exacerbate dissociation and are not recommended. The inclusion of the dissociative subtype of PTSD in DSM–5 and emerging evidence about how those who dissociate respond to treatment will help guide future research and treatment planning for individuals with PTSD who dissociate.

Psychosis

Definition and Prevalence

Psychotic symptoms, which include hallucinations, delusions, catatonia, or thought disorders, can range from mild to severe and can be present in several Axis I disorders, including schizophrenia, depression with psychotic features, and Type I bipolar affective disorder. Psychotic symptoms such as hallucinations are reported with PTSD in up to 50% of cases (Anketell et al., 2010). In veteran populations, between 16% and 48% of individuals with Axis I disorders involving psychosis have comorbid PTSD (Álvarez et al., 2012).

Considerations

Psychotic-like symptoms (hallucinations, paranoia) that are secondary to traumas associated with PTSD may appear to overlap with primary psychotic symptoms more typically associated with psychotic disorders. An individual with PTSD may experience significant hypervigilance, a decreased sense of safety, and pervasive lack of trust, but these should be distinguished from paranoia associated with impaired reality testing in which individuals may fear or believe "everyone" is out to get them or that others are talking about or judging them in some way. It should be noted, however, that the distinction between hypervigilance and paranoia can at times be difficult to make. Olfactory hallucinations may be more commonly associated with PTSD, for example, when a veteran still perceives aversive smells reminiscent of those encountered on the battlefield, such as burning oil or blood. Bizarre delusions or delusions of reference are not associated with PTSD.

Implications

Thorough assessment of thought content, context, and insight can help clinicians differentiate between psychotic disorders and psychosis secondary to PTSD. Individuals with psychotic disorders such as schizophrenia who have experienced traumatic events may weave content from prior traumatic experiences into delusional thought processes. In addition, family history of significant mood or psychotic disorders is important to assess to provide information about genetic predisposition. Preliminary studies suggest that EBTs for PTSD can be helpful for someone with psychotic symptoms (see van Minnen, Harned, Zoellner, & Mills, 2012), but as of yet little is known about the type and severity of psychosis for which EBTs might be contraindicated. Treatment with medication should be directed at symptomatology, and psychotic symptoms in PTSD that have not resolved after EBTs should be treated with antipsychotic medication. Antipsychotics have not been shown to be effective in treating PTSD without psychosis (Ipser & Stein, 2012). Given the significant metabolic risks associated with antipsychotic medications and the lack of efficacy of these medications in the absence of comorbid psychotic disorders, accurate diagnosis is key. Treatment of comorbid PTSD in patients with severe mental illness requires a team-based approach, full medical workup for new-onset psychosis, and specialty referral when available.

Borderline Personality Disorder

Definition and Prevalence

BPD is defined by a constellation of severely impairing traits involving marked affective instability, poor sense of self, transient stress-related paranoid ideations, dissociative-like symptoms, reckless or self-injurious behavior, feelings of emptiness, and unstable interpersonal relationships. As many as 58% of individuals with BPD meet criteria for PTSD, a rate much higher than that seen in the general population (Zanarini et al., 1998). Rates of BPD in PTSD have been shown to be about 24% (Pagura et al., 2010).

Considerations

Early childhood trauma is common among individuals with BPD. The high incidence of child abuse in BPD patients, up to 91%, has prompted theories that BPD more accurately represents a complex and chronic form of PTSD. It should be noted, however, that BPD as a diagnosis is highly comorbid with a variety of other Axis I and Axis II disorders. Therefore, conceptualizing BPD simply as a complex form of PTSD may represent an oversimplification of the social, psychological, genetic, and environmental factors involved in the development of BPD. A key distinction between BPD and PTSD is the long-standing and enduring patterns of these traits in individuals with BPD. Patients with PTSD would typically demonstrate a history of fairly stable premorbid relationships and functioning before their trauma. However, it may not be possible to draw this distinction with individuals who developed PTSD in early childhood.

Implications

Thorough assessment of BPD with a particular focus on safety is needed to determine an appropriate treatment plan. Individuals with BPD without serious self-injurious behaviors have been shown to benefit from EBTs for PTSD, such as PE (see van Minnen et al., 2012). However, for severe forms of BPD involving self-injurious behaviors or high suicide risk, integrated treatment for BPD and PTSD has been recommended. For example, a stepped approach that first focuses on safety, coping skills, or emotional regulation and then on trauma processing has been shown to be efficacious for individuals with extreme mood dysregulation or self-harming tendencies (e.g., Cloitre et al., 2010). Dialectical behavior therapy (DBT) is an EBT for BPD, and studies are in progress to evaluate combined DBT and PE protocols (Harned, Korslund, Foa, & Linehan, 2012). A review by van Minnen and colleagues (2012) showed insufficient evidence to offer PE to individuals who have made recent (past 2 months) suicide attempts. Although pharmacotherapy may not significantly address overall severity of BPD, antidepressants may address mood and anxiety symptoms associated with both BPD and PTSD. Mood stabilizers and second-generation antipsychotics may target specific core symptoms associated with BPD (Lieb, Völlm, Rücker, Timmer, & Stoffers, 2010). Medications should therefore target specific symptoms, although effect on overall severity in complex BPD presentations may be limited.

Eating Disorders

Definition and Prevalence

Eating disorders such as anorexia nervosa, bulimia nervosa, and binge-eating disorder (BED) are characterized by extreme attitudes and behaviors relating to weight, body image and food consumption that can result in significant emotional distress, serious health complications, or even death. The limited number of studies examining the prevalence of PTSD among individuals with eating disorders report a comorbidity ranging from 11% to 52% (Gleaves, Eberenz, & May, 1998; Turnbull, Troop, & Treasure, 1997) with particularly high rates of PTSD seen in individuals with bulimia (up to 3 times higher) compared with those with anorexia alone (Kaye, Bulik, Thornton, Barbarich, & Masters, 2004). Among women, the National Women's Study (Dansky, Brewerton, Kilpatrick, & O'Neil, 1997) found a lifetime prevalence of PTSD of 36.9% in women with bulimia nervosa and 21% in BED, whereas the lifetime PTSD prevalence was only 11.8% in participants without an eating disorder.

Considerations

PTSD and eating disorders share some common risk factors. For example, trauma during childhood development such as physical, sexual, or emotional abuse increases the risk of later eating disorders. Women sexual assault survivors also manifest increased rates of eating-disordered behaviors, as do women veterans with trauma exposure related to combat (Mitchell, Wells, Mendes, & Resick, 2012). Binge-eating behaviors are frequently associated with impulsivity and attempts to regulate negative affective states and thus might be used by individuals with PTSD to regulate anxiety and negative affect. Additionally, such behaviors may enable some trauma survivors with PTSD with means to escape self-awareness, and for some, bingeing or purging behavior may produce a dissociative-type state.

Implications

A thorough evaluation can help determine whether eating-disordered behaviors are secondary to trauma versus more primary eating disorder behaviors.

Careful assessment of attitudes relating to weight, food consumption, purging behaviors, and exercise should be undertaken, and a food log is useful to evaluate severity. Currently, there are no clear guidelines for treatment of comorbid PTSD and eating disorders. For non–life-threatening eating disorder presentations, PTSD psychotherapy has been shown to alleviate ED behaviors that occur primarily in response to trauma triggers or function as a form of avoidance (Mitchell et al., 2012). However, someone who engages in behaviors or is at a weight that may cause medical complications needs more intensive treatment for ED in combination with PTSD treatment. Even among individuals whose eating disorder started in the context of PTSD, additional therapy may be needed for specific disordered eating attitudes and behaviors. Eating disorders have the highest mortality rates of any psychiatric disorder, and severe cases require specialized treatment with multidisciplinary care (social work, family therapy, nutrition, psychiatrist, psychologist). Research has shown some antidepressants, mood stabilizers, and antipsychotic medications can target mood or anxiety symptoms and reduce obsessional thoughts about food or body image, although results are modest. Antidepressants such as fluoxetine (Prozac), which is currently the only selective serotonin reuptake inhibitor approved to treat bulimia nervosa, may assist in reducing binge-eating and purging behaviors and alleviate symptoms of anxiety and depression in PTSD, typically at higher doses. Bupropion (Wellbutrin) should be avoided in individuals with bulimia or anorexia. The anticonvulsant topiramate (Topamax) has been found to reduce binge-eating episodes, along with a resultant small decrease in body weight, in binge-eating disorder.

RECOMMENDATIONS FOR CLINICAL PRACTICE AND FUTURE RESEARCH

When present along with PTSD, many conditions and symptoms can complicate assessment, treatment, and, in some cases, prognosis. The literature points to the following as areas that require special attention in clinical and research practice.

Safety

Across problems and disorders, safety is a primary determinant for treatment planning. Regular and detailed safety assessments throughout treatment can alert clinicians to the possibility of increasing symptoms or decompensation during treatment. Imminent safety concerns, whether in regard to medical issues, aggression, or self-harm, require immediate attention. Whether EBTs for PTSD should be delivered in an integrated fashion while addressing disorder-specific safety issues or postponed until safety issues are stabilized is a question that requires further research. Such decisions are generally made on a case-by-case basis depending on the patient's level of risk. When deciding on a course of treatment, it is important to consider that many patients who were previously believed to be too unstable for EBTs can in fact benefit from these treatments (van Minnen et al., 2012).

Assessment

The high rates of comorbidity with other disorders and associated problems highlight the importance of a thorough standardized initial assessment using validated diagnostic instruments. Assessing which symptoms or conditions are the most impairing can help guide treatment planning. Conversely, PTSD is sometimes overlooked in some cases in which other highly impairing disorders (e.g., psychosis, BPD) are present. Such oversight could negatively affect treatment outcomes because failure to treat comorbid PTSD has been shown to impede recovery from other disorders. Additional research is needed to help guide clinicians in distinguishing seemingly overlapping symptoms (e.g., guardedness vs. paranoia) when trying to differentiate symptoms of PTSD from other disorders.

Treatment

Treating challenging presentations of PTSD necessitates a multidisciplinary team approach. Often, a well-coordinated combination of best practice psychotherapy, psychopharmacologic approaches, and case management is needed to maximize recovery. The literature suggests that in many cases, treatment of PTSD can lead to reduction in symptoms of both PTSD and other disorders. This is encouraging in that EBT for PTSD can reduce symptoms in as little as 6 to 12 weeks. However, this review also shows that for challenging cases, especially when safety is a concern, integrative treatments of both PTSD and other co-occurring disorders and problems are warranted. These treatments generally help patients understand why their disorders commonly co-occur, address safety issues, teach emotional regulation and coping skills, and then transition into trauma processing. At what point during such treatments it is appropriate to begin trauma processing remains an empirical question. Such protocols are typically longer than standard EBTs for PTSD, and evidence is needed to guide the appropriate length of treatment. As of yet, there are few randomized clinical trials of integrated treatments for PTSD and specific comorbidities to guide clinicians. Questions about appropriate level of care also remain. Residential treatment offers a level of structure and intensity that may benefit individuals with challenging presentations, but at which stage of treatment someone is best able to benefit from residential care remains to be answered. Studies that combine psychotherapy and pharmacology are also needed to develop best practices for treating challenging presentations of PTSD.

REFERENCES

Adetunji, B., Mathews, M., Williams, A., Budar, K., Mathews, M., Mahmud, J., & Osinowo, T. (2005). Use of antipsychotics in the treatment of posttraumatic stress disorder. *Psychiatry, 2*, 43–47.

Álvarez, M.-J., Roura, P., Foguet, Q., Osés, A., Solà, J., & Arrufat, F.-X. (2012). Posttraumatic stress disorder comorbidity and clinical implications in patients with severe mental illness. *Journal of Nervous and Mental Disease, 200*, 549–552. doi:10.1097/NMD.0b013e318257cdf2

American Psychiatric Association. (2013). *Diagnostic and statistical manual of mental disorders* (5th ed.). Washington, DC: Author.

Anketell, C., Dorahy, M. J., Shannon, M., Elder, R., Hamilton, G., Corry, M., . . . O'Rawe, B. (2010). An exploratory analysis of voice hearing in chronic

PTSD: Potential associated mechanisms. *Journal of Trauma & Dissociation, 11,* 93–107. doi:10.1080/15299730903143600

Bushman, B. J., & Huesmann, L. R. (2010). Aggression. In S. T. Fiske, D. T. Gilbert, & G. Lindzey (Eds.), *Handbook of social psychology* (5th ed., pp. 833–863). New York, NY: Wiley.

Carlson, E., Dalenberg, C., & McDade-Montez, E. (2012). Dissociation in posttraumatic stress disorder: Recommendations for modifying the diagnostic criteria for PTSD. *Psychological Trauma: Theory, Research, Practice, and Policy, 4,* 551–559.

Cloitre, M., Stovall-McClough, K. C., Nooner, K., Zorbas, P., Cherry, S., Jackson, C. L., . . . Petkova, E. (2010). Treatment for PTSD related to childhood abuse: A randomized controlled trial. *The American Journal of Psychiatry, 167,* 915–924. doi:10.1176/appi.ajp.2010.09081247

Dansky, B. S., Brewerton, T. D., Kilpatrick, D. G., & O'Neil, P. M. (1997). The National Women's Study: Relationship of victimization and posttraumatic stress disorder to bulimia nervosa. *International Journal of Eating Disorders, 21,* 213–228. doi:10.1002/(SICI)1098-108X(199704)21:33.0.CO;2-N

Elbogen, E. B., Johnson, S. C., Wagner, H. R., Newton, V. M., & Beckham, J. C. (2012). Financial well-being and postdeployment adjustment among Iraq and Afghanistan war veterans. *Military Medicine, 177,* 669–675. doi:10.7205/MILMED-D-11-00388

Elbogen, E. B., Wagner, H. R., Calhoun, P. S., Fuller, S. R., & Kinneer, P. M. (2010). Correlates of anger and hostility among Iraq and Afghanistan war veterans. *The American Journal of Psychiatry, 167,* 1051. doi:10.1176/appi.ajp.2010.09050739

Gleaves, D. H., Eberenz, K. P., & May, M. C. (1998). Scope and significance of posttraumatic symptomatology among women hospitalized for an eating disorder. *International Journal of Eating Disorders, 24,* 147–156. doi:10.1002/(SICI)1098-108X(199809)24:2<147::AID-EAT4>3.0.CO;2-E

Hagenaars, M. A., van Minnen, A., & Hoogduin, K. A. (2010). The impact of dissociation and depression on the efficacy of prolonged exposure treatment for PTSD. *Behaviour Research and Therapy, 48,* 19–27. doi:10.1016/j.brat.2009.09.001

Harned, M. S., Korslund, K. E., Foa, E. B., & Linehan, M. M. (2012). Treating PTSD in suicidal and self-injuring women with borderline personality disorder: Development and preliminary evaluation of a dialectical behavior therapy prolonged exposure protocol. *Behaviour Research and Therapy, 50,* 381–386. doi:10.1016/j.brat.2012.02.011

Hunter, E. C., Sierra, M., & David, A. S. (2004). The epidemiology of depersonalisation and derealisation. *Social Psychiatry and Psychiatric Epidemiology, 39,* 9–18. doi:10.1007/s00127-004-0701-4

Ipser, J. C., & Stein, D. J. (2012). Evidence-based pharmacotherapy of posttraumatic stress disorder (PTSD). *International Journal of Neuropsychopharmacology, 15*, 825–840. doi:10.1017/S1461145711001209

Jakupcak, M., Conybeare, D., Phelps, L., Hunt, S., Holmes, H. A., Felker, B., . . . McFall, M. E. (2007). Anger, hostility, and aggression among Iraq and Afghanistan war veterans reporting PTSD and subthreshold PTSD. *Journal of Traumatic Stress, 20*, 945–954. doi:10.1002/jts.20258

Kaye, W. H., Bulik, C. M., Thornton, L., Barbarich, N., & Masters, K. (2004). Comorbidity of anxiety disorders with anorexia and bulimia nervosa. *American Journal of Psychiatry, 161*, 2215–2221. doi:10.1176/appi.ajp.161.12.2215

Kessler, R. C., Sonnega, A., Bromet, E., Hughes, M., & Nelson, C. B. (1995). Posttraumatic stress disorder in the national comorbidity survey. *Archives of General Psychiatry, 52*, 1048. doi:10.1001/archpsyc.1995.03950240066012

Lanius, R. A., Brand, B., Vermetten, E., Frewen, P. A., & Spiegel, D. (2012). The dissociative subtype of posttraumatic stress disorder: Rationale, clinical and neurobiological evidence, and implications. *Depression and Anxiety, 29*, 701–708. doi:10.1002/da.21889

Lieb, K., Völlm, B., Rücker, G., Timmer, A., & Stoffers, J. M. (2010). Pharmacotherapy for borderline personality disorder: Cochrane systematic review of randomised trials. *The British Journal of Psychiatry, 196*, 4–12. doi:10.1192/bjp.bp.108.062984

Marshall, A. D., Martin, E. K., Warfield, G. A., Doron-Lamarca, S., Niles, B. L., & Taft, C. T. (2010). The impact of antisocial personality characteristics on anger management treatment for veterans with PTSD. *Psychological Trauma: Theory, Research, Practice, and Policy, 2*, 224–231. doi:10.1037/a0019890

Mitchell, K. S., Wells, S. Y., Mendes, A., & Resick, P. A. (2012). Treatment improves symptoms shared by PTSD and disordered eating. *Journal of Traumatic Stress, 25*, 535–542. doi:10.1002/jts.21737

Pagura, J., Stein, M. B., Bolton, J. M., Cox, B. J., Grant, B., & Sareen, J. (2010). Comorbidity of borderline personality disorder and posttraumatic stress disorder in the U.S. population. *Journal of Psychiatric Research, 44*, 1190–1198. doi:10.1016/j.jpsychires.2010.04.016

Resick, P. A., Suvak, M. K., Johnides, B. D., Mitchell, K. S., & Iverson, K. M. (2012). The impact of dissociation on PTSD treatment with cognitive processing therapy. *Depression and Anxiety, 29*, 718–730. doi:10.1002/da.21938

Taft, C. T., Weatherill, R. P., Woodward, H. E., Pinto, L. A., Watkins, L. E., Miller, M. W., & Dekel, R. (2009). Intimate partner and general aggression perpetration among combat veterans presenting to a posttraumatic stress disorder clinic. *American Journal of Orthopsychiatry, 79,* 461–468. doi:10.1037/ a0016657

Turnbull, S. J., Troop, N. A., & Treasure, J. L. (1997). The prevalence of post-traumatic stress disorder and its relation to childhood adversity in subjects with eating disorders. *European Eating Disorders Review, 5,* 270–277. doi:10.1002/(SICI)1099-0968(199712)5:4<270::AID-ERV212>3.0.CO;2-3

van Minnen, A., Harned, M. S., Zoellner, L., & Mills, K. (2012). Examining potential contraindications for prolonged exposure therapy for PTSD. *European Journal of Psychotraumatology, 3.* doi:10.3402/ejpt.v3i0.18805

Zanarini, M. C., Frankenburg, F. R., Dubo, E. D., Sickel, A. E., Trikha, A., Levin, A., & Reynolds, V. (1998). Axis I comorbidity of borderline personality disorder. *The American Journal of Psychiatry, 155,* 1733–1739.

Zlotnick, C., Begin, A., Shea, M. T., Pearlstein, T., Simpson, E., & Costello, E. (1994). The relationship between characteristics of sexual abuse and dissociative experiences. *Comprehensive Psychiatry, 35,* 465–470. doi:10.1016/0010-440X(94)90230-5

Index

Acamprosate, 137, 138
Acute stress, 16
ADIS (Anxiety Disorders Interview Schedule for *DSM*), 45
Adolescents, 108, 165
Adrenal gland, 13
Affect, 93, 105, 170
Agency for Healthcare Research and Quality (AHRQ), 56, 61
Aggression, 38, 73, 165–166
Alcohol use, 46, 80, 136–138
Alcohol Use Disorders Identification Test (AUDIT), 136
Allopregnanolone and pregnanolone (ALLO), 16, 17
Allostatic load, 17
Alpha-2 adrenergic agonists, 61
Alpha-antagonists, 155
Alprazolam, 71, 77, 81
Altruism, 24
American Academy of Sleep Medicine, 124, 125
American Psychiatric Association, 78, 109
American Psychological Association (APA), 22
Amitriptyline, 56

Amygdala
    effects of CBT treatments on, 110
    in neurocircuitry of PTSD, 17
    and resilience, 23, 24
    in species-specific defense response, 9, 11–15
Anorexia nervosa, 172
Anticonvulsant treatment of PTSD
    costs of, 95–96
    limited data supporting use of, 89
    overview, 92–93
    research on, 61
Antidepressant management of PTSD, 55–64
    with comorbid borderline personality disorder, 171
    with comorbid eating disorders, 173
    with co-occurring insomnia, 125
    with mirtazapine/nefazodone/ trazodone, 59
    with nonserotonergic agents, 60–63
    for older adults, 155
    research on, 55–56
    and resilience, 25
    with SSRIs and SNRIs, 56–59
    with TCAs and MAOIs, 56, 59–60

179

INDEX

Antipsychotic treatment of PTSD
    for aggression symptoms, 166
    case example, 94–95
    with comorbid borderline personality disorder, 171
    with comorbid eating disorders, 173
    with co-occurring insomnia, 125–126
    costs of, 95–96
    limited data supporting use of, 89, 170
    for older adults, 154, 155
    overview, 62, 90–91
    and sleep problems, 80
Antisocial personality disorder, 45
Anxiety
    assessment of, 45, 46
    benzodiazepines for treatment of, 71, 72. *See also* Benzodiazepine treatments, for management of PTSD
    and insomnia, 120
    psychosocial training for reducing, 27
Anxiety disorders, 36, 37
Anxiety Disorders Interview Schedule for *DSM* (ADIS), 45
Anxiolytics. *See* Benzodiazepine treatments, for management of PTSD
APA (American Psychological Association), 22
Apoptosis, 15
Assessment
    for challenging presentations of PTSD, 174
    of eating disorders, 173
    of insomnia, 127
    of PTSD. *See* Posttraumatic stress disorder assessment and diagnosis
    of resilience, 22

Atypical antipsychotics. *See* Antipsychotic treatment of PTSD
AUDIT (Alcohol Use Disorders Identification Test), 136
Augmentation strategies (pharmacotherapy), 6
Autonomic nervous system, 9
Avoidance symptoms
    in *DSM* criteria, 36–37, 58
    in *ICD* criteria, 38
    pharmacotherapy options for treating, 89, 155
Axis I comorbidities. *See* Comorbid disorders

Barbiturates, 72
Basolateral nucleus of the amygdala (BLA), 9, 11, 13
BED (binge-eating disorder), 172, 173
Behavioral changes, for insomnia treatment, 122
Behavioral observations, 39
Benzodiazepine treatments, for management of PTSD, 71–83
    case study, 82–83
    and concurrent psychotherapy, 109
    with co-occurring insomnia, 126
    currently favored treatments, 81–82
    and dissociation, 168
    evidence-based use of, 76–78
    guideline recommendations, 77–79
    for older adults, 155
    potential risks with, 62, 72–76
    prescribing recommendations, 79–80
Berenz, E. C., 142
Best practice guidelines (BPGs), 102, 109–110
Beta-adrenergic antagonists, 60–61
Beta-blockers, 26
Bienvenu, O. J., 78
Binge-eating disorder (BED), 172, 173

Bipolar affective disorder, 169
BLA (basolateral nucleus of the amygdala), 9, 11, 13
Blain, L. M., 106
Borderline personality disorder (BPD), 164, 170–171
Bottom-up processes, with pharmacotherapy, 5
BPD (borderline personality disorder), 164, 170–171
BPGs (best practice guidelines), 102, 109–110
Bulimia nervosa, 172
Buprenorphine, 140–141
Bupropion, 139, 173

Caffeine use, 80
Calhoun, P. S., 38
Candidate genes, implicated in PTSD, 12
Cannabis, 137
Cannon, Walter, 13
CAPS. *See* Clinician Administered PTSD Scale
Cardiovascular disease, 120
Catatonia, 169
Catecholamines, 16
CBT–I (cognitive behavioral therapy for insomnia), 79–81, 124–125
CBTs. *See* Cognitive behavioral therapies
Central nucleus of the amygdala, 13, 14
Challenging presentations of PTSD, 163–174
  aggression, 165–166
  assessment with, 174
  with borderline personality disorder, 164, 170–171
  differentiating PTSD symptoms from comorbid conditions, 89–90
  dissociation, 164, 167–168
  eating disorders, 172–173

  psychosis, 169–170
  safety considerations for, 171, 174
  treatment considerations for, 174–175
Chappuis, C., 106
Chard, K. M., 106
Child abuse and childhood trauma, 23, 36, 106, 170–172
Children, 6, 108
Chronic stress
  cortisol dysregulation in, 15
  effects of, 21
Clinician Administered PTSD Scale (CAPS)
  and anticonvulsant treatment of PTSD, 92, 93
  and antipsychotic treatment of PTSD, 90, 91
  overview, 40, 43–44
Cloitre, M., 168
Clonazepam, 71, 77
Coffey, S. F., 142
Cognitive behavioral therapies (CBTs), 101–111
  addressing symptoms through, 93
  for aggression, 166
  and benzodiazepine treatment, 75, 81
  brain mechanisms of, 5
  cognitive processing therapy. *See* Cognitive processing therapy
  early interventions with, 28–29
  evidence-based, 103–108, 125
  eye movement desensitization and reprocessing (EMDR), 107, 123–124
  imagery rehearsal therapy, 107–108, 124
  and insomnia, 79–81, 122–125
  for older adults, 156
  overview, 102
  and pharmacotherapy, 63, 79, 108–111

181

prolonged exposure therapy.
See Prolonged exposure
therapy
for sleep, 93. *See also* Cognitive
behavioral therapy for
insomnia
stress inoculation training, 26–27,
103
for substance use disorder treatment, 141, 142
Cognitive behavioral therapy for
insomnia (CBT–I), 79–81,
124–125
Cognitive flexibility, 24
Cognitive functioning, 74, 154, 157
Cognitive processing therapy (CPT),
105–106
addressing symptoms through, 93
benzodiazepines' interference
with, 76
fear extinction with, 12
outcomes with, 156, 157
for treatment of co-occurring
SUDs, 143
for treatment of dissociation, 168
Community resilience, 24–25
Comorbid disorders, 45–47, 163–164.
See also Challenging presentations of PTSD; *specific disorders, e.g.:* Insomnia,
119–133, Substance Use
Disorder, 135–150
Comprehensive Solder and Family
Fitness (CSF), 26
Concurrent Treatment of PTSD and
Substance Use Disorders Using
Prolonged Exposure (COPE),
142–143
Connor Davidson Scale, 22
Coping skills, 24, 27
Corticotropin-release hormone
(CRH), 14, 17

Corticotropin-release hormone
antagonists, 25
Cortisol, 15
CPT. *See* Cognitive processing
therapy
CRH (corticotropin-release
hormone), 14, 17
CSF (Comprehensive Solder and
Family Fitness), 26
Cytokines, 16, 17

DA. *See* Dopamine
Davydow, D. S., 78
DBT (dialectical behavior therapy),
171
DDRI–2 (Deployment Risk and
Resilience Inventory—2), 40
Decision making, shared, 6
Dehydroepiandrosterone (DHEA),
15, 17, 25
Delusions, 169
Dementia, 74, 154
Depersonalization, 167
Deployment Risk and Resilience
Inventory—2 (DDRI–2), 40
Depression
CBT for treatment of, 109
measures for assessment of, 46
psychosocial training for
reducing, 27
with psychotic features, 169
Derealization, 167
Desai, S. V., 78
Developmental factors, in resilience,
23
DHEA (dehydroepiandrosterone), 15,
17, 25
Diagnosis, of PTSD. *See* Posttraumatic
stress disorder assessment and
diagnosis
*Diagnostic and Statistical Manual of
Mental Disorders (DSM–III)*, 72

INDEX

Diagnostic and Statistical Manual of Mental Disorders (DSM–IV)
  assessing comorbid conditions using criteria from, 45
  and diagnostic interview measures for PTSD, 43, 44
  overview of PTSD criteria, 36–38
  and self-report PTSD symptom measures, 41–42

Diagnostic and Statistical Manual of Mental Disorders (DSM–5)
  assessing comorbid conditions using criteria from, 45
  and diagnostic interview measures for PTSD, 43, 44
  dissociative subtype of PTSD in, 167, 168
  overview of PTSD criteria, 36–39
  and prevalence rates, 47, 165
  and self-report PTSD symptom measures, 41–42
  and SSRI treatment of PTSD, 58
  substance use disorders in, 136

Diagnostic interview measures
  for assessing comorbid conditions, 45
  for assessing PTSD, 39, 43–44

Dialectical behavior therapy (DBT), 171
Diazepam, 71
Dispositional Resilience Scales, 22
Dissociation, 164, 167–168
Disulfiram, 137, 138
Divalproex, 92, 93, 96
DoD (U.S. Department of Defense), 78, 123
Dopamine (DA)
  gene variants affecting, 22
  and resilience, 22, 24
  in species-specific defense response, 11, 13–14

DSM. *See Diagnostic and Statistical Manual of Mental Disorders*
Duke Global Rating for PTSD, 92
Duloxetine, 71

Early intervention, 28–29
Eating disorders, 45, 172–173
ELS (Evaluation of Lifetime Stressors), 40–41
Elwood, L., 106
EMDR (eye movement desensitization and reprocessing), 107, 123–124
Emotional processing theory, 103–104
Emotional resilience, 26
Emotion regulation, 24, 164, 167
Escitalopram, 71, 72, 79
Eszopiclone, 62, 126
Ethical principles, 24
Evaluation of Lifetime Stressors (ELS), 40–41
Evidence-based treatments
  for aggression, 166
  with benzodiazepines, 76–78
  for borderline personality disorder, 171
  cognitive behavioral therapies, 103–108, 123
  for dissociation, 168
  integrated delivery of, 174
  for psychotic symptoms, 170
  symptom improvement with, 175
Exposure therapy
  benzodiazepines' interference with, 76
  prolonged. *See* Prolonged exposure therapy
  support for use of, 156–157
Eye movement desensitization and reprocessing (EMDR), 107, 123–124

Families, 26
FDA (U.S. Food and Drug Administration), 56, 71–72
Fear conditioning, 12, 15, 77
Fear extinction, 12, 15, 76
Fear responses
　and benzodiazepines, 76, 77
　in prolonged exposure, 103–104
　and serotonin, 14
　in stress inoculation training, 103
Fight-or-flight response, 13. *See also* Human stress response
5-HT. *See* Serotonin
Fletcher, T., 106
Fluoxetine, 57, 173
Foa, E. B., 103, 104
Functional impairment
　assessment of, 45–47
　in *DSM* criteria, 37
　in *ICD* criteria, 39

GABA (gamma-aminobutyric acid)
　anticonvulsants' effect on, 92
　in species-specific defense response, 11, 15, 16
Galovski, T. E., 106, 108
Gelpin, E., 78
Genetic factors, in resilience, 22–23
Gifford, J. M., 78
Glucocorticoids, 16, 17
Glutamate
　anticonvulsants' effect on, 92
　in species-specific defense response, 11, 13
Group therapy, 156

Habituation, 168
Hallucinations, 169
Hardiness Training, 26–27
Health, 152–153
Hippocampus
　in neurocircuitry of PTSD, 17
　and resilience, 23, 24
　in species-specific defense response, 11, 13, 15
Houle, T., 106
HPA axis. *See* Hypothalamic–pituitary–adrenocortical axis
Human stress response, 9–17
　adaptive function of, 9
　intervention and treatment implications, 17
　map of, 10
　neurohormones/neuropeptides involved in, 14–16
　neurotransmitters involved in, 13–14
　overview, 10, 12–13
　relevance of, to PTSD, 16–17
　research on resilience's role in, 25
Hyperarousal symptoms
　antidepressants for treatment of, 59
　antipsychotics for treatment of, 89, 90
　benzodiazepines for treatment of, 72, 155
　in *DSM* criteria, 37, 38
　in *ICD* criteria, 39
Hypervigilance, 169
Hypothalamic–pituitary–adrenocortical (HPA) axis
　corticotropin-release hormone in, 14
　cortisol and dehydroepiandrosterone in, 15
　and dysregulation in PTSD, 17
　gene variants affecting, 22
　negative feedback on, 16
　and resilience, 22–25
　in species-specific defense response, 9, 10, 12

ICD–11 (*International Classification of Diseases, 11th Edition*), 38–39, 44, 136

INDEX

Imagery rehearsal therapy (IRT), 107–108, 124, 125
Imipramine, 56
Immune factors
    with benzodiazepine usage, 73
    in resilience, 23
    in species-specific defense response, 16
Impact of Events Scale—Revised, 42
Information processing behaviors, 9, 12
Insomnia, 119–128
    algorithm for assessment and treatment of, 127
    behavioral and lifestyle changes for treatment of, 122
    benzodiazepines for treatment of, 72, 74, 78
    and cognitive behavioral therapies, 79–81, 123–125
    conditions aggravating, 121–122
    consequences of, 120
    eye movement desensitization and reprocessing (EMDR) for treatment of, 123–124
    imagery rehearsal therapy for treatment of, 107, 124, 125
    and nightmares, 120–121
    pharmacological treatment of, 125–126
Institute of Medicine (IOM), 56, 57
Insula, 110
International Classification of Diseases, 11th Edition (ICD–11), 38–39, 44, 136
International Society for Traumatic Stress Studies, 78, 123
Interpersonal regulation, 93
Interpersonal relationships, 170
Interview measures, diagnostic. *See* Diagnostic interview measures
Intrusion symptoms, 58
Inventory of Psychosocial Functioning (IPF), 46
IOM (Institute of Medicine), 56, 57
Irritability, 38
IRT (imagery rehearsal therapy), 107–108, 124, 125

Kaysen, D., 111, 143
Kozak, M. J., 103

Lamotrigine, 61, 92, 96
Learned Optimism (CBT approach), 27
Life Events Checklist (LEC), 39–40
Lifestyle changes, for insomnia treatment, 122
Litz, B. T., 26
Locus coeruleus, 14
Lorazepam, 71

MAOIs (monoamine oxidase inhibitors), 56, 59–60
McCauley, J. L., 142
Medication. *See* Pharmacotherapy
Meditation, mindfulness, 27
Meichenbaum, D., 103
Memory
    affect associated with, 105
    overconsolidation of traumatic memories, 25–26
    in species-specific defense response, 11–12
Meta-chlorophenylpiperazine, 14
Methadone, 140
Millennium Cohort Study, 121
Miller, M. W., 38
Mindfulness meditation training, 27
MINI-International Neuropsychiatric Interview (MINI), 45
Minnesota Multiphasic Personality Inventory—2, 42
Mirtazapine, 59, 79
Mississippi Scale for Combat-Related PTSD, 42
Monoamine oxidase inhibitors (MAOIs), 56, 59–60

Mood disorders, 45
Mood stabilizers, 155, 171, 173
Moral principles, 24
Morphine, 26
Mott, J. M., 106

Naloxone, 141
Naltrexone, 137, 138, 140, 141, 144–145
Nash, W. P., 26
National Institute for Clinical Excellence (NICE), 56, 57
National Women's Study, 172
Navy and Marine Corps Combat and Operational Stress First Aid model, 26
NE. See Norepinephrine
Needham, D. M., 78
Nefazodone, 59, 125
Network Support Therapy, 27
Neurobiological factors, in resilience, 23–25
Neuroendocrine system, 9, 14
Neurogenesis, 15
Neurohormones, 14–16
Neuropeptides, 14–16
Neuropeptide Y (NPY), 15, 17, 25
Neurotoxicity, 15
Neurotransmitters, 13–14
NICE (National Institute for Clinical Excellence), 56
Nicotine replacement therapy (NRT), 138–139
Nightmares
  imagery rehearsal therapy for treatment of, 107
  and insomnia, 120–121, 124
  pharmacotherapy options for treatment of, 60, 80, 90
Norepinephrine (NE), 11, 13, 17, 22. See also Serotonin-norepinephrine reuptake inhibitors
Norris, F. H., 24

NPY (neuropeptide Y), 15, 17, 25
NRT (nicotine replacement therapy), 138–139
Numbing symptoms, 36–37, 59

Olanzapine, 90, 91, 125–126
Older adults with PTSD, 151–158
  benzodiazepine use by, 73, 74, 80, 82
  and longitudinal course of PTSD, 153–154
  pharmacological treatments, 154–155
  psychotherapy treatments, 110, 156–158
  statistics on, 152–153
Olfactory hallucinations, 169
Operation Enduring Freedom veterans, 76, 121
Operation Iraqi Freedom veterans, 76, 121
Opioids, 76, 82, 137, 140–141
Oxycodone, 76

Panic disorder, 81
Paranoid ideation, 170
Paroxetine, 56, 168
Partial responders, 6
Patient Health Questionnaire (PHQ), 45–46
PCL (PTSD Checklist), 41–42, 90
PDS (Posttraumatic Dialogistic Scale), 42
Peritrauma risk factors, 35, 36
Persistent negative appraisals, 37
Persistent negative mood, 37
Personality disorders, 166. See also Borderline personality disorder
PE therapy. See Prolonged exposure therapy
PFC. See Prefrontal cortex

INDEX

Pharmacotherapy. *See also specific treatment types, e.g.:* Antidepressant management of PTSD
  bottom-up processes with, 5
  for children, 6
  and cognitive behavioral therapies, 63, 79, 108–111
  for comorbid psychotic symptoms, 170
  future directions for research on, 5–6
  for older adults with PTSD, 154–155
  and resilience, 23–26
  for treatment of co-occurring SUDs, 144–145
  for treatment of insomnia, 125–126
Phenelzine, 59
PHQ (Patient Health Questionnaire), 45–46
Physical fitness, 24, 26
Pietrzak, R. H., 152
Polysedative use, 76
Posttrauma social support, 36
Posttraumatic Dialogistic Scale (PDS), 42
Posttraumatic stress disorder (PTSD). *See also specific headings*
  pathophysiology of, 5
  prevalence of, 38, 47, 152, 165
  validity/utility of diagnosis of, 3
Posttraumatic stress disorder assessment and diagnosis, 35–47
  of comorbidity, 45–47
  diagnostic interview measures for, 39, 43–44
  DSM criteria for, 36–39
  of functional impairment, 45–47
  and risk factors, 35–36
  self-report symptom measures for, 39, 41–43
  trauma exposure measures for, 39–41
  validity/utility of diagnosis of, 3
Prazosin
  for treating comorbid SUDs, 145
  for treating co-occurring insomnia, 79, 80, 91, 126, 128
  for treatment of nightmares, 60, 90, 95
  for treatment of PTSD in older adults, 154
Prefrontal cortex (PFC)
  in neurocircuitry of PTSD, 17
  psychosocial training for enhancing activation in, 27
  and resilience, 23, 24
  in species-specific defense response, 11, 13–15
Pregnanolone, 16, 17
Present-centered therapy, 104
Pretraumatic risk factors, 35
Prevalence, of PTSD, 38, 47, 152, 165
Primary Care Posttraumatic Stress Disorder screen, 41
Proinflammatory cytokines, 16, 17
Prolonged exposure (PE) therapy
  addressing symptoms through, 93
  concurrent pharmacotherapy and, 108–109
  efficacy of, 93
  outcomes with, 156, 157
  overview, 103–104
  for treatment of borderline personality disorder, 171
  for treatment of dissociation, 168
Propranolol, 60–61
Psychoeducation, 103
Psychological First Aid, 28
Psychopathy, 166
Psychosis, comorbid, 169–170
Psychosocial functioning, 24, 46

Psychosocial training, 26–27
Psychotherapy
    cognitive behavioral. *See* Cognitive behavioral therapies
    mechanisms of action in, 5
    for older adults with PTSD, 110, 156–158
    as primary treatment modality for PTSD, 93
    for treating co-occurring substance use disorders, 141–145
    for treating insomnia, 122–125
Psychotic disorders, 45
PTSD. *See* Posttraumatic stress disorder
PTSD Checklist (PCL), 41–42, 90
PTSD Clinical Practice Guideline Workgroup, 79
PTSD Symptom Scale Interview, 44

Quetiapine, 125–126

Ramesh, V., 120
Raphe nuclei, 11, 14
Reckless behavior, 38
Reexperiencing symptoms
    in *DSM* criteria, 36
    in *ICD* criteria, 38
    pharmacotherapy options for treating, 89, 155
Relationships, interpersonal, 170
Relaxation training, 156
Resick, Patricia, 105, 168
Resilience, 21–29
    assessment of, 22
    community factors, 24–25
    defined, 21–22
    Deployment Risk and Resilience Inventory–2, 40
    developmental factors, 23
    early intervention for fostering, 28–29
    genetic factors, 22–23
    neurobiological factors, 23–25
    neurobiological/pharmacological strategies for enhancing, 25–26
    psychosocial factors, 24
    psychosocial training for enhancing, 26–27
    and species-specific defense response, 15, 16
    and threat appraisal, 12
Response to Stressful Experiences, 22
Richardson, G., 108
Risk factors, for PTSD, 35–36
Risperidone, 90–91, 95
Rothbaum, B. O., 104, 108

Safety considerations, 171, 174
Schizophrenia, 169
Schneier, F. R., 109
SCID–I (Structured Clinical Interview for the *DSM–IV–TR* Axis I Disorders), 45
Selective serotonin reuptake inhibitors (SSRIs)
    as anxiolytics, 71, 79
    concurrent use with CBT, 79
    as first-line agents for PTSD treatment, 89
    limited efficacy in treating PTSD, 14
    management of PTSD with, 56–59
    support for use in PTSD treatment, 109
    for treatment of anxiety disorders, 71–72
    for treatment of eating disorders, 173
    for treatment of insomnia, 125
Self-destructive behavior, 38
Self-efficacy, 24, 27, 29
Self-report symptom measures
    for comorbid disorders, 45–46

INDEX

for PTSD assessment/diagnosis, 39, 41–43
for substance use disorders, 136
Serotonin (5-HT)
  and ALLO activation, 16
  drugs inhibiting reuptake of. *See* Selective serotonin reuptake inhibitors; Serotonin-norepinephrine reuptake inhibitors
  gene variants affecting, 22–23
  in species-specific defense response, 11, 14, 17
Serotonin-norepinephrine reuptake inhibitors (SNRIs)
  as anxiolytics, 71, 79
  as first-line agents for PTSD treatment, 89
  management of PTSD with, 56–59
  support for use in PTSD treatment, 109
  for treatment of anxiety disorders, 71–72
  for treatment of insomnia, 125
Sertraline
  as anxiolytic, 71
  and cognitive behavioral therapies, 104, 108–109
  FDA approval for treatment of PTSD, 56, 57
  for treating co-occurring insomnia, 145
Shapiro, Francine, 107
Shared decision-making model, 6
Short Posttraumatic Stress Disorder Rating Interview, 41
Short Screening Scale for PTSD, 41
SI–PTSD (Structured Interview for PTSD), 44
SIT (stress inoculation training), 26–27, 103
Skeletal muscle behaviors, 9

Skill development, for resilience, 24, 29
Sleep and sleep problems. *See also* Insomnia
  antipsychotics for treatment of, 90, 91
  cognitive behavioral therapies for, 93. *See also* Cognitive behavioral therapy for insomnia
  effects of benzodiazepines on, 74, 76
Sleep hygiene, 80, 122
Smoking, 80, 137–140, 144
SNRIs. *See* Serotonin-norepinephrine reuptake inhibitors
Social support
  as factor in resilience, 24, 26, 27
  posttrauma, 36
Socratic questioning, 105
Spirituality, 24, 26
SSDR (species-specific defense response), 9–14, 16–17. *See also* Human stress response
SSRIs. *See* Selective serotonin reuptake inhibitors
Startle Physiological Arousal, Anger, and Numbness Scale, 41
Steenkamp, M. M., 26
Stimulant use, 137
Stress. *See also* Human stress response
  acute, 16
  chronic, 15, 21
Stress First Aid, 28
Stress inoculation training (SIT), 26–27, 103
Structured Clinical Interview for the *DSM–IV–TR* Axis I Disorders (SCID–I), 45
Structured Interview for PTSD (SI–PTSD), 44
"Stuck points" (cognitive processing therapy), 105

Substance use disorders (SUDs), co-occurring, 135–146
  alcohol, 46, 80, 136–138
  benzodiazepines, 78, 82
  clinical management of, 145–146
  combined pharmacotherapy/psychotherapy for treating, 144–145
  diagnosis of, 136–137
  and insomnia, 121, 122
  measures for assessment of, 45
  opioids, 76, 82, 137, 140–141
  psychotherapy for treating, 141–145
  single-medication approach with, 145
  tobacco, 80, 137–140, 144
  treatment strategy for, 137
Suicidality, 45, 137
Sympathetic nervous system, 13, 23–25
Symptom Checklist 90—Revised, 42
Symptom severity, 42, 45

Tapering, 72, 80, 81, 82, 83, 94, 138, 155
TCAs. See Tricyclic antidepressants
TF–CBT (trauma-focused cognitive behavioral therapy), 108
Therapy. See Psychotherapy
Thought disorders, 169
Threat appraisal, 12
Tiagabine, 61, 92, 93, 96
TNF (tumor necrosis factor)-alpha gene, 120
Tobacco, 80, 137–140, 144
Top-down processes
  with cognitive behavioral therapy, 5
  in species-specific defense response, 11
Topiramate
  evidence supporting use of, 61, 95, 96
  symptom reduction with, 92
  for treatment of co-occurring eating disorders, 173
  for treatment of co-occurring SUDs, 137, 138, 145
Torchalla, I., 142, 143
Trauma exposure measures, 39–41
Trauma-focused cognitive behavioral therapy (TF–CBT), 108
Trauma History Questionnaire, 40
Traumatic brain injury, 74, 80, 82, 121–122
Traumatic Events Questionnaire, 40
Traumatic Life Events Questionnaire, 40
Trazodone, 59, 79, 125
Treatment outcomes, 5
Tricyclic antidepressants (TCAs)
  management of PTSD with, 56, 59–60
  for older adults, 155
  for treatment of sleep problems, 79
Tumor necrosis factor (TNF)-alpha gene, 120
Type I bipolar affective disorder, 169

U.S. Department of Defense (DoD), 78, 123
U.S. Department of Veterans Affairs (VA), 78, 123
U.S. Food and Drug Administration (FDA), 56, 71–72

VA (U.S. Department of Veterans Affairs), 78, 123
Valproate, 61
Van Dam, D., 142
Van Minnen, A., 171
Varenicline, 139–140
Venlafaxine, 56–58, 71
Verbal memory, 157
Veterans Health Administration, 111

Veterans with PTSD
   aggression in, 165
   anticonvulsants for treatment of, 73–76, 79
   antidepressants for treatment of, 56, 58–60
   benzodiazepine for treatment of, 73–76, 79
   and cognitive processing therapy, 106
   comorbid psychosis in, 169
   dissociative features of, 167
   eating disorders in, 172
   and exposure therapy, 157
   insomnia and sleep disturbances in, 77, 121
   prevalence of, 38, 152
   substance use by, 139
Vigilance, 121, 169
Violence, 165, 166. *See also* Aggression
Visuospatial function, 120

Weight gain, 120
WHO (World Health Organization), 56
WHODAS (World Health Organization Disability Assessment Schedule), 46–47
Williams, A. M., 108
Woodward, S., 121
Working memory, 13
World Health Assembly, 38
World Health Organization (WHO), 56
World Health Organization Disability Assessment Schedule (WHODAS), 46–47

Zaleplon, 126
Zolpidem, 62, 126

About the Editors

Nancy C. Bernardy, PhD, is a biological and clinical research psychologist who has served for the past 6 years as the director of the PTSD Mentoring Program for the Executive Division of the U.S. Department of Veterans Affairs' National Center for PTSD. She also serves as an associate director for clinical networking at the center. She is an assistant professor of psychiatry at the Geisel School of Medicine at Dartmouth. Dr. Bernardy has 20 years of experience as a clinician and researcher, with approximately 35 publications. She is a member of the American Psychological Association and the International Society for Traumatic Stress Studies, and she serves on numerous national research, education, and policy committees for the Department of Veterans Affairs.

Matthew J. Friedman, MD, PhD, served for 25 years as executive director of the U.S. Department of Veterans Affairs' National Center for PTSD. He recently stepped down to become a senior advisor to the center. In addition, he is a professor of psychiatry and of pharmacology and toxicology at the Geisel School of Medicine at Dartmouth. He has over 40 years of experience as a clinician and researcher, with approximately 300 publications, including 27 books. Dr. Friedman is a Distinguished Lifetime Fellow of the American Psychiatric Association, past president of the International Society for Traumatic Stress Studies, chair of the American Psychiatric Association's *DSM-5* PTSD Work Group, and chair of the Scientific Advisory Board of the Anxiety Disorders Association of America. He has served on many national research, education, and policy committees. Past honors include the International Society for Traumatic Stress Studies Lifetime Achievement Award in 1999 and the Public Advocacy Award in 2009. Dr. Friedman was a finalist for the 2011 Samuel J. Heyman Service to America Medal.